W9-BXH-345

Virus Diseases and the Nervous System

Virus Diseases and the Nervous System

A Symposium edited by

C. W. M. Whitty

Department of Neurology

J. T. Hughes

Department of Neuropathology

F. O. MacCallum

Department of Virology

United Oxford Hospitals

Blackwell Scientific Publications

Oxford and Edinburgh

© BLACKWELL SCIENTIFIC PUBLICATIONS LTD 1969

*This book is copyright. It may not
be reproduced by any means in whole
or in part without permission.
Application with regard to copyright
should be addressed to the publishers.*

SBN 632 05970 2

FIRST PUBLISHED 1969

616.8
V821

Printed in Great Britain by
ADLARD AND SON LTD DORKING
and bound by
THE KEMP HALL BINDERY, OXFORD

Contents

22 631

*Joint authors of the paper, not attending the symposium.

Viruses and Malignant Disease of the Nervous System
CHAIRMAN: DR S. NEVIN

General Discussion
CHAIRMAN: DR F. O. MACCALLUM

Participants

Dr Ingrid Allen *Institute of Pathology, Queen's University, Belfast.*

Dr June Almeida *Department of Virology, Postgraduate Medical School, London, W.12.*

Dr M. Alpers *Department of Microbiology, School of Medicine, Victoria Square, Perth, W. Australia.*

Mrs Elisabeth Beck *Department of Neuropathology, Institute of Psychiatry, Maudsley Hospital, London.*

Professor P. B. Beeson *Nuffield Department of Clinical Medicine, The Radcliffe Infirmary, Oxford.*

Dr L. van Bogaert *Instituut Bunge, Filip Williotstraat, 59, Berchem-Antwerpen, Belgium.*

Dr B. D. Bower *Paediatric Department, The Radcliffe Infirmary, Oxford.*

Dr E. M. Brett *The Hospital for Sick Children, Great Ormond Street, London.*

Dr Betty Brownell *Department of Neuropathology, The Radcliffe Infirmary, Oxford.*

Professor Melville Calvin *University of Berkeley, California, U.S.A.*

Dr J. A. N. Corsellis *Department of Neuropathology, Runwell Hospital, Wickford, Essex.*

Dr P. B. Croft *Neurology Department, Whittington Hospital, London.*

P. M. Daniel* *Department of Neuropathology, Institute of Psychiatry, The Maudsley Hospital, London.*

Professor C. D. Darlington *Botany School, South Parks Road, Oxford.*

Dr A. D. Dayan *Department of Pathology, Hospital for Sick Children, Great Ormond Street, London.*

*Joint authors of the paper, not attending the symposium.

Professor G. W. Dick   *Bland-Sutton Institute of Pathology, Middlesex Hospital, London.*

Dr C. C. Draper   *Wellcome Research Laboratories, Beckenham, Kent.*

Dr C. Earl   *The National Hospital for Nervous Diseases, Queen Square, London.*

Dr D. C. Gajdusek*   *Laboratory of Slow, Latent and Temperate Virus Infections, National Institute of Neurological Diseases, Bethesda, Maryland, U.S.A.*

Dr A. Galbraith   *Geigy (U.K.) Ltd., Pharmaceuticals Division, Macclesfield, Cheshire.*

Dr C. J. Gibbs*   *Laboratory of Slow, Latent and Temperate Virus Infections, National Institute of Neurological Diseases, Bethesda, Maryland, U.S.A.*

Dr D. A. Haig   *Department of Microbiology, Institute for Research on Animal Diseases, Compton, Newbury, Berks.*

Dr D. G. F. Harriman   *Neuropathology Department, General Infirmary, Leeds.*

Professor Henry Harris   *Sir William Dunn School of Pathology, Oxford.*

Dr R. E. Hope-Simpson   *Epidemiological Research Unit, Dyer Street, Cirencester.*

Dr R. L. Hewer   *Department of Neurology, The Churchill Hospital, Oxford.*

Dr J. T. Hughes   *Department of Neuropathology, The Radcliffe Infirmary, Oxford.*

Dr G. D. Hunter   *Institute for Research on Animal Diseases, Compton, Newbury, Berks.*

Dr Ralph Johnson   *Department of Neurology, Churchill Hospital, Oxford.*

Professor Sir Hans Krebs   *Metabolic Research Unit, The Radcliffe Infirmary, Oxford.*

Dr N. J. Legg   *National Hospital for Nervous Diseases, Queen Square, London.*

Dr F. O. MacCallum   *Virology Department, The Radcliffe Infirmary, Oxford.*

Dr E. D. McDonnell   *Department of Biochemistry, Tennis Court Road, Cambridge.*

Dr A. M. R. Mackenzie   *Virology Department, The Radcliffe Infirmary, Oxford.*

Professor W. H. McMenemey   *Department of Neuropathology, Maida Vale Hospital, London.*

Dr W. B. Matthews   *Department of Neurology, Manchester Royal Infirmary.*

Dr S. Nevin   *Maida Vale Hospital, London.*

Dr R. E. Offord   *Department of Zoology, University Museum, Oxford.*

Dr D. R. Oppenheimer   *Department of Neuropathology, The Radcliffe Infirmary, Oxford.*

Dr J. M. Oxbury   *Department of Neurology, The Churchill Hospital, Oxford.*

Dr C. Pallis   *Department of Neurology, Postgraduate Medical School, London, W.12.*

Dr H. B. Parry   *Nuffield Institute for Medical Research, Oxford.*

Mr J. Pennybacker   *Department of Neurosurgery, The Radcliffe Infirmary, Oxford.*

Mr J. M. Potter   *Department of Neurosurgery, The Radcliffe Infirmary, Oxford.*

Dr A. H. T. Robb-Smith   *The Gibson Laboratories, The Radcliffe Infirmary, Oxford.*

Dr D. R. Redman   *Royal Hospital, Sheffield.*

Dr Honor V. Smith   *Department of Neurology, The Churchill Hospital, Oxford.*

Dr J. M. K. Spalding   *Department of Neurology, The Radcliffe Infirmary, Oxford.*

Dr J. D. Spillane   *Department of Neurology, Cardiff Royal Infirmary, Cardiff.*

Mr C. Stolkin   *Osler House, The Radcliffe Infirmary, Oxford.*

Dr A. H. Tomlinson   *Public Health Laboratory, The Radcliffe Infirmary, Oxford.*

Dr D. A. J. Tyrrell   *Clinical Research Centre Laboratories, National Institute for Medical Research, Mill Hill, London.*

Dr V. Udall   *Wellcome Research Laboratory, Beckenham, Kent.*

Professor H. Urich   *Bernhard Baron Institute of Pathology, London Hospital, Whitechapel, London.*

Dr Roy Vollum   *Lincoln College, Oxford.*

Professor A. P. Waterson   *Department of Virology, Postgraduate Medical School, London. W.12.*

Dr H. E. Webb   *St. Thomas's Hospital, London.*

Dr C. E. C. Wells   *Department of Neurology, Cardiff Royal Infirmary, Cardiff.*

Dr C. W. M. Whitty   *Department of Neurology, The Radcliffe Infirmary, Oxford.*

Dr Marcia Wilkinson   *Elizabeth Garrett Anderson Hospital, London.*

Mr A. J. Ruff   *Symposia Officer, Geigy (U.K.) Limited, Pharmaceuticals Division, Macclesfield, Cheshire.*

Mrs Margaret Raynes   *Geigy (U.K.) Limited, Pharmaceuticals Division.*

Preface

Recent rapid advances in knowledge of some aspects of virus diseases of the nervous system and particularly the application of new ideas on the mechanism of virus infections and the nature and role of the infective agent, prompted the organizing of this symposium. Geigy (U.K.) Ltd., Pharmaceuticals Division gave us generous financial support and we are grateful to them, and particularly to Dr Alan Galbraith and Mr A.J. Ruff for their help. Mrs Margaret Raynes' work in transcribing the proceedings was also invaluable. The symposium was held in the attractive setting of Somerville College and our thanks are due to the Principal and Governing Body for allowing us to meet there.

Radcliffe Infirmary,   C.W.M.W.

United Oxford Hospitals.   J.T.H.

July, 1968   F.O.M.

Acute Virus Diseases of the Nervous System

Chairman
F. O. MacCallum

Introduction

F. O. MacCallum

When my colleagues asked me if I would help them to organize this
meeting my immediate reaction was that there had been so many
recent meetings, lectures, papers and editorials on infection with so-
called slow viruses, subacute sclerosing panencephalitis and acute
encephalitis that there would be little interest in another two-day
discussion. However, as we talked over and around the subject during
several sessions, and one or two more papers and editorials appeared,
it became increasingly obvious that there were numerous gaps in communication of available information in all our sub-specialities quite
apart from the ignorance which we all share on various aspects of the
pathogenesis of some of the diseases which are on our programme.
In my naïvety, I was slightly surprised at the failure of communication
but I realize that my virological colleagues and I in the United Oxford
Hospitals are fortunate in that almost every week we are consulted about
the investigation of one or more patients with a variety of apparent
CNS diseases.

I will quote only one simple, but to the virologists, obvious example
of this lack of communication or understanding between some interested parties in the field under discussion this morning—acute encephalitis. An annotation or leading article in one of the weekly journals
in March 1968, referring to a case of encephalitis in a recent paper on
some Coxsackie B5 infections stated, 'Coxsackie virus may have been
missed in the past because these viruses are not often considered as a
cause of virus encephalitis.' No virology laboratory worthy of its name
has worked in the manner this statement implies for about ten years.
If the writer had said that Coxsackie viruses were considered to be an
uncommon cause of encephalitis that would have been a different
matter. The advice on investigation of aetiology of encephalitis has been
for some years now to collect throat swabs or washings, faeces, CSF
and blood and nowadays also ventricle fluid and even brain biopsy
when available; also of course, convalescent serum for antibodies.
The specimens are inoculated into several types of tissue culture which

between them should support growth with accompanying cytopathic effect of polio-viruses, echoviruses, Coxsackie B and several Coxsackie A viruses, reo viruses, mumps, herpes simplex, zoster, measles and cytomegaloviruses. New born mice are inoculated for isolation of those Coxsackie viruses which do not produce a cytopathic effect in the tissue cultures, and of arboviruses. This may be done immediately or after waiting for results of tissue culture. Nowadays it is probable that immunofluorescence will be used on cells in CSF or smears or tissues. The point is that although one may have a suspicion of some particular agent it is virtually impossible to differentiate between the signs and symptoms caused by the numerous possible agents, and with rare exceptions you must investigate with this in mind and not with any fixed preconceived idea, even if some particular virus is prevalent at the time.

We arranged the programme in its present form for two reasons. First, because of our very small staff and lack of facilities for large scale experiments in animals we have been concerned particularly with diagnosis and possible treatment of acute encephalitis and we thought that if some of the local team took the floor first after Dr Tyrrell, it would provide an opportunity for the visitors to settle in and also digest some of Dr Tyrrell's remarks.

Second and equally, this arrangement seemed a suitable sequence. It would probably be more logical for acute encephalitis to be followed by persistent latent and chronic infections, which would include subacute sclerosing leucoencephalitis, but of course we shall be mentioning persistent latent infection when discussing herpes simplex infection. We thought that discussion about the slow viruses deserved the longer time and it was better to attack it freshly after lunch. The topics for the third session are obviously still on the fringe and may be related to any of today's topics or possibly not at all. I believed they provide a focus for fascinating speculation though I understand that some neurologists are doubtful whether the subjects merit the attention and time we have allotted to them.

While considering the time interval between infection and the onset of definable symptoms of the CNS and how the discussion might go, I remembered a meeting of the Neuropathology Club about 1950 in which subacute inclusion body encephalitis was being discussed because five or six cases in London and the South East had been recently investigated by several of us. The late Professor Greenfield with his wealth of experience stated that this condition existed only in the subacute or chronic state, at which I, as a virologist, expostulated that there must be an acute stage. It appears that we were both partly correct.

This disease and the recent observations on it seem to me to provide a useful pointer for the direction in which studies of suspected virus diseases in the CNS should be pursued in the United Kingdom. It is easy to have fixed ideas of a disease one has seen for a long time and perhaps fail to react to a new situation such as electron microscopy presents. On the other hand it is also very easy to believe, rather than hope, that new techniques such as electron microscopy and fluorescence are going to solve all our problems immediately. In the hands of experts, such as Dr Almeida and Professor Waterson, the electron microscope is a useful tool, but virus-like bodies seen in the electron microscope may still to some extent have the same place as intranuclear inclusions had in stained tissue many years ago. I believe that we need more active and progressive cooperation between clinical experience and youthful enthusiasm and technical know-how in this field. Collaboration between Queen Square hospital and Great Ormond Street, the new Virology Department at Hammersmith and the London Hospital, and work in Professor Dick's department at the Middlesex and in the group at Newcastle are indications that this is underway.

One of the invited virologists who unfortunately is missing as he is working at present in California, wrote to me before his departure—'The trouble is that most of the interesting work on viruses and the CNS is going on in other countries.' Obviously he was not including the work on scrapie and I would like to think that there is work going on in relation to diseases in man of which he is unaware. Possibly Dr Alpers and other visitors will tell us just how much is going on already and how far we are behind.

A number of the neurologists whom we approached to participate replied that they had nothing of value to contribute but wished to attend. As obvious virus disease is responsible for only a small proportion of the patients they see, this attitude is quite understandable; I believe that there has been only one case of subacute sclerosing panencephalitis in Oxford in seven years. With this in mind we have tried to allow ample time for discussion and we hope that the selected speakers will stimulate your thought processes as well as each others and we are counting on your active, not passive, participation.

Virus Behaviour and the Cell

D. A. J. Tyrrell

Viruses are basically very small organisms in which the genetic information is encoded either in DNA or RNA. They can replicate only inside
cells, for only in these can they find the biochemical machinery they
require for the synthesis of new components. There are viruses of
plants and bacteria as well as the vertebrates but this summary is
concerned primarily with animal viruses growing in vetebrate cells.

Types of virus particle

Viruses are classified at the moment by the salient features of their
structure and some of these are set out in Table 1. In all cases the nucleic
acid is found inside the virus particle and is associated with protein.
The protein units may form a cage or shell in which they are arranged
with cubic symmetry in relation to each other and the particle as a whole
(Fig. 1). In every case so far studied the particles have been more or

TABLE I. CHARACTERISTICS OF SOME IMPORTANT VIRUSES

Name	Symmetry	Nucleic acid	Diameter (mμ)	Essential lipid* (ether labile)
Adeno	Cubic	DNA	70	—
Picorna (Enteroviruses and rhinoviruses)	Cubic	RNA	30	—
Herpes	Cubic	DNA	120–130	+
Papova (Warts, polyoma SV40)	Cubic	DNA	45	—
Myxo (and paramyxo)	Helical	RNA	100–200	+

*Viruses which have cell components as essential units of their structure are made
non-infectious by exposure to ether and other lipid solvents.

7

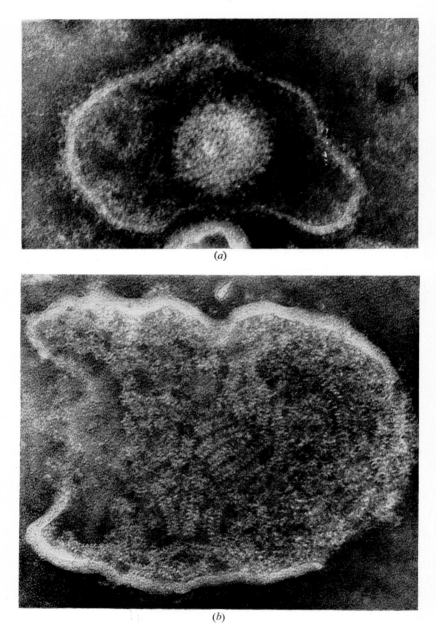

(a)

(b)

less icosahedrical in shape. In other viruses the nucleic acid is arranged as a spiral with associated protein, and the whole is enclosed within an envelope composed of a complex of components derived from the host and others specified by the virus. Such a virus is said to have helical symmetry. Viruses possess either RNA or DNA—never both—and this may also be used in classification. Another fundamental point in structure is the amount of nucleic acid and the number and size of protein units, and these are in a general way reflected in the size of the particle, which is usually expressed as the diameter.

Multiplication of a cytolytic virus
Since there are so many different sorts of viruses and host cells the interaction between them takes many forms. However it will be helpful to start by describing some of the features of the multiplication of a typical small RNA virus, an enterovirus such as the poliovirus (Fig. 2). The virus particle is carried or diffuses to the cell surface where it is anchored by electrostatic forces while an ill-understood active process, perhaps related to pinocytosis, brings it into the cytoplasm. At this stage the protein coat is dissolved, probably by cellular enzymes, and the RNA enters the cytoplasm. Here it specifies the production of a polymerase, which, using the RNA as a template and nucleotides from the cell pool, induces the synthesis of more RNA strands (Fig. 3); a double stranded form being produced at an intermediate stage. This RNA then acts as a messenger and induces the cell ribosomes to produce a protein which forms the capsid or protein coat of the new virus particles, and probably other proteins which are involved in the assembly of complete virus particles. At an early stage the virus may also do something, perhaps synthesize another protein, which inhibits the synthesis by the cell of its own nucleic acids and proteins (Fig. 4) and, in the best studied examples, by the time virus synthesis is nearing completion, the cell rounds up, its surface seems to 'boil', and virus particles are shed into the surrounding medium. These virus particles then spread in body fluids through the circulation or through the outer environment to other cells which may in turn be destroyed. Not all

---

FIGURE I. Examples of cubic and helical symmetry in virus structure:

(a) a herpes virus showing the icosahedral arrangements of 'hollow' subunits which forms the outer coat or capsid of the particle.

(b) the internal component or nucleocapsid of a parainfluenza virus. (Photographs by Dr June D. Almeida.)

body cells are equally susceptible to the virus and it is the pattern of susceptibility which determines the pathogenesis of the disease. Thus, the poliovirus multiplies freely in the cells of the alimentary tract, to some extent in the upper respiratory tract and not at all in the kidney, and this determines the fact that infection is spread primarily by the

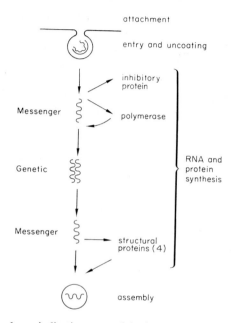

FIGURE 2. A scheme indicating some of the features of the multiplication of enterovirus, such as poliovirus. On the left are shown the type of function exercised by the RNA strand at each stage. See text for further details.

faecal-oral route. However, the virus also multiplies in anterior horn cells and those of the brain stem, and this determines the occurrence of paralytic disease, which affects a proportion of subjects who have viraemia during an alimentary tract infection. Poliomyelitis is the end result of infection with a virus which has a complete growth cycle and is destructive or cytolytic.

Multiplication of some other viruses
Other viruses vary from this pattern in one way or the other. For example adenoviruses are DNA viruses and they are bigger. They also

replicate primarily in the nucleus and induce the formation of a number of proteins, some of which are known to be enzymes. As in the normal cell, the virus DNA induces specific RNA which enters the cytoplasm and induces the formation of proteins which are assembled into particles around the DNA 'cores' which form in the nucleus. The cell rounds up but does not disintegrate and the virus remains in the cell, protected from the external environment; when the cell finally dies the particles in the nucleus are released. In certain conditions, such as the infection of an 'unsuitable' cell or the lack of an amino acid, complete adenovirus may not be made, although some of the specific virus proteins are. In circumstances of this sort the presence of another virus in the cell, a helper virus, such as the virus SV40, may in monkey kidney cells enable the adenovirus to multiply completely; in a similar way the adenovirus may act as a helper for small DNA viruses called adeno-associated or satellite viruses, which cannot multiply in uninfected cells and which therefore spread in partnership with a normal adeno-virus. If virus does not multiply completely it may nevertheless have profound effects on cell metabolism; in particular it may induce malig-nant transformation as will be described later. The virus in transformed cells is replicating in step with the cell itself and may continue to specify the production of some 'early' proteins, and also 'new' surface antigens which may be responsible for transplantation immune reactions. It is unlikely that such viruses become incorporated into the cell chromo-some in exactly the same way as temperate phages but nevertheless such infected cells resemble in a number of ways lysogenic bacteria. Viruses may also produce specific proteins and complete virus in cells which are apparently functioning normally. One example is the virus SV40; the DNA of this virus is produced in the cell nucleus, and com-pleted particles must pass through the cytoplasm to be shed, and yet in monkey kidney cultures prepared from certain species there may be little or no cell destruction (usually called cytopathic effect or CPE), although in the cells of other species such as the vervet monkey, there may be extensive vacuolation of the cytoplasm.

Viruses such as myxoviruses are formed at cell membranes, and the outer membrane of the virus includes host cell membrane components as well as virus protein. This membrane is wrapped around a coiled coil of virus nucleic acid as a virus bud or filament is formed. This occurs at the surface of the cell in the case of influenza viruses. Para-myxoviruses like NDV may form at the membranes of cytoplasmic vesicles, and this seems to be the usual site for completion of the particles

D. A. J. Tyrrell

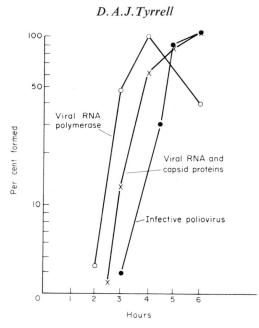

FIGURE 3. Growth curve of poliovirus, indicating the times at which components mentioned in Figure 2 are synthesized.

of certain RNA tumour viruses, arboviruses and the viruses of the avian-infectious-bronchitis group. In these cells there may be either severe damage to the cells or very little.

In some cases, for example the parainfluenza or measles virus, large amounts of the internal helical component may accumulate in the cytoplasm, as though there was an incoordination of production or assembly of the virus particles; there are, in fact, laboratory model systems in which little or no measles or parainfluenza 2 virus is produced although most of the cells of the culture are full of virus antigen.

The cellular response to virus infections is, in many of its aspects, ill-understood. Cytoplasmic inclusions are often seen and may represent deposits of viral nucleic acid or protein, as just mentioned. Basic and acidophilic inclusions in the nuclei of cells infected with adenoviruses are sites in which virus nucleic acid and protein accumulate, and sometimes virus protein may crystallize out. However, as in the case of herpes virus infection, inclusions may be largely fixation and staining artefacts formed during the histological processing of an infected cell.

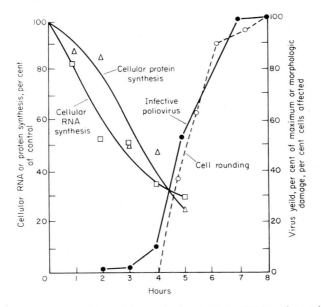

FIGURE 4. The inhibition of the synthesis of cellular RNA and protein by poliovirus. (Figures 3 and 4 reproduced by permission of I. Tamm and the Rockefeller University Press.)

In addition, cells in which normal synthetic processes have been inhibited by the virus will die just like cells treated with chemical inhibitors such as actinomycin D. On the other hand, it has recently been shown that the appearance of degenerative changes may depend on whether there is damage to lysosomes. If these are damaged the hydrolytic enzymes they contain may be released into the cytoplasm and cause autolysis. If damage due to proteolysis is controlled or repaired they might enter the nucleus and cause chromosomal damage by disrupting molecules of DNA.

Other factors in the pathogenesis of virus diseases
In many cases the interferon system, which may be thought of as a defence mechanism against the entry of foreign genetic information into the cell, is triggered by virus multiplication. The presence of double stranded nucleic acid in the early stages of virus replication stimulates the production of the protein interferon. This then enters adjacent cells and stimulates the formation of another protein; this protein

apparently affects the ribosomes so that the information carried on a 'foreign' virus messenger RNA does not become translated into new protein molecules. This effect is remarkable, for it is so specific that the cells own RNA and protein synthesis proceeds normally, while it is completely protected from the harmful effects of the synthesis of a wide range of viruses.

When specific virus proteins are shed from cells and circulate in the body, they are recognized as 'foreign' and so stimulate the production of antibodies. Antibodies directed against the internal components of viruses have in general, little effect on the virus particle although their detection by a complement-fixation test may be a useful diagnostic test. However antibodies which react with the surface of a virus usually render it non-infectious—they are called virus-neutralizing antibodies and play an important role in resisting and eliminating infections. They can only inactivate extracellular virus particles, since they cannot penetrate the intact cell membrane.

Finally we must make a brief mention of some other possible reactions between viruses, cells and immune systems. Animals congenitally infected with lymphocytic choriomeningitis virus are tolerant to viral antigens which are treated as foreign proteins and induce the formation of antibodies by animals which are infected later in life. There are also examples of hypersensitivity reactions to viruses; these are probably responsible for much of the cell tissue response in the accelerated or 'immune' response to vaccination against smallpox and also for the fatal encephalitis which occurs in mice which are infected with lymphocytic choriomeningitis virus in adult life rather than in infancy. Cutaneous hypersensitivity to mumps and herpes viruses has also been shown in man and some sort of hypersensitivity may lie behind the severe reactions to measles seen in children vaccinated with some killed vaccines

The 'new' virus antigens which may appear at cell surfaces induce specific cell-mediated transplantation immunity to neoplastic cells, but it is possible that similar reactions may from time to time take place with infected but untransformed cells. This possibility would bear further investigation as also would the exact roles of the different species of gamma globulins. It is known that γG, γA and γM molecules can all neutralize viruses, but early antibodies against certain viruses particularly herpes, may require complement to do so with maximum efficiency. Some bird antibodies may not neutralize, or may even enhance infectivity. In some circumstances antibodies directed against the cell surface rather than against the virus may protect it against infection.

Finally, since so many viruses enter the body by mucous surfaces it is obvious that the recently discovered local production of secretory antibody may be very important in protecting against infection. The γA formed in the respiratory tract can neutralize viruses, appears after virus infection and may be correlated with immunity to experimental infections with respiratory viruses.

Although this represents a cursory review of the wide field of modern virology it does, I hope, include most of the important principles which are required for the understanding of more detailed papers which follow.

REFERENCES

General virology
HORSFALL F.L. Jr & TAMM I. (1965) *Viral and Rickettsial Infections of Man*, 4th Ed. London.
ANDREWES C.H. & PEREIRA H.G. (1964) *Viruses of Vertebrates*, 2nd Ed. London.

Interferon
FINTER N. (ed.) (1966) *Interferons*, Amsterdam.

Importance of local antibody
SMITH C.B., PURCELL R.H., BELLANTI J.A. & CHANOCK R.M. (1966) Protective effect of antibody to parainfluenza virus. *New Engl. J. Med.* **275**, 1145–1152.
ROSSEN R.D. MORGAN C., HSU K.C., BUTLER W.T. & ROSE H.M. (1968) Localisation of 11S external secretary IgA by immunofluorescence in Tissue lining oral and respiratory passages in man. *J. Immunol.* **100**, 706–717.

Clinical Aspects of Herpes Simplex Encephalitis

J. M. Potter

It is an honour for a surgeon to be asked to talk on the clinical aspects of herpes simplex encephalitis, and I shall confine my brief general review to those aspects that strike a neurosurgeon and have been within my own experience and that of Mr Pennybacker and others in the Department of Neurological Surgery here in Oxford.

It is because these cases have been referred to us that surgical biopsy has been performed. And it was because Dr MacCallum had joined us that it became possible, while the patients were still alive, to learn for certain (MacCallum, Potter & Edwards, 1964) that the condition which we already knew as acute necrotizing, inclusion-body or haemorrhagic encephalitis, could be due to the herpes simplex virus.

Fred MacCallum has been a great stimulus to us. Before he came, we were not much interested in these cases. As junior staff, I remember, we would sporadically dispatch various specimens (although not brain biopsies, I think) to distant parts—a procedure that came to be known as 'sending letters to Father Christmas'. Nothing happened!—and as far as we were concerned, it all seemed rather a waste of time, or at least what would currently be called a failure of communication. Now it is interesting; if not yet rewarding in a way a clinician likes to be rewarded—with a cure.

In the past, these patients usually came to us with a presumptive diagnosis of brain abscess or tumour. Nowadays, greater awareness of this form of encephalitis has encouraged the correct diagnosis to be made earlier, although I should stress now—as I will again later— that, for as long as I can remember, cases actually of brain *abscess*, *tumour* and *tuberculous meningitis* have been referred to us with an initial diagnosis of *encephalitis*, but for the exclusion of those remediable conditions, notably abscess and tuberculous meningitis, which can of course be cured if treated appropriately and *in good time*.

This is of course *the* task for the clinician, verification of the diagnosis beyond all reasonable doubt: in these cases (apart from those of tuberculous meningitis), the process consists essentially of clinical localization of the main lesion, supported and refined by appropriate radiological investigation and then, usually, cannulation of the affected

17

area of the brain, when aspiration produces pus, blood or histologically recognizable neoplastic tissue—or encephalitis from which tissue the herpes simplex virus may be obtained.

Our patients with herpetic encephalitis have all had clinical evidence of *infection*: fever, malaise, headache and leucocytosis—features which may of course be common also to brain abscess and tuberculous meningitis—and occasionally to neoplasm if, say, the terminal stage of chest infection has been reached. The symptoms and signs that follow may be equally non-specific: drowsiness, confusion, stupor, coma, epileptic fits, meningism, and lateralizing and focal signs referable, in these cases, particularly to one or other temporal region.

The CSF has only occasionally been normal, as it may be in cases of tumour and abscess. Commonly, there has been a pleocytosis of up to 100 or 200 white cells, mostly or exclusively lymphocytes; a raised protein content, but always normal sugar, and no organisms on the Gram film or from culture. This lymphocytic picture may be seen also when a malignant tumour is necrotic and close to the CSF pathways, and tumour cells may easily be taken for lymphocytes; and the same lymphocytic picture is very occasionally seen following cerebral haemorrhage. In tuberculous meningitis, there is more likely to be a reduction in the sugar content and one would hope to find tubercle bacilli—but these characteristics may of course be absent. Similarly—and Dr Honor Smith will go into all this much more expertly later—the CSF reaction to an acute abscess may be a lymphocytic one, with no organisms seen or grown.

Thus far, a *firm clinical diagnosis* is not within our power, and it is necessary to resort to carotid angiography (we have not yet tested the isotope brain-scanning method for these particular cases). Angiography reveals an avascular mass, mainly in the temporal lobe, which might be, again, an abscess, a neoplasm, a haematoma, an infarct—or a swollen area of necrotizing encephalitis. A burr-hole biopsy decides which, and not only excludes a remediable lesion but is the only means of positively identifying the virus at this stage of the illness.

The outlook for the confirmed cases of herpes simplex encephalitis has been a gloomy one. With few exceptions, those surviving have been demented to a severe degree. This has presumably resulted from widespread necrosis in the temporal region, probably medially and to some extent bilaterally; and if any therapeutic agent is to be effective it would, again I say *presumably*, have to be given systemically to reach these parts *before necrosis occurs*.

But it seems that we in neurosurgical departments are sent these cases only because of the severity of the brain disturbance *already produced by the necrotizing process*, which by then probably cannot be undone. It is for this reason that we do not feel that surgical decompression (which we have performed twice) is a particularly relevant or promising form of treatment. What appears to me to be needed—and we shall no doubt hear more about iodoxuridine—is an effective, non-toxic agent which can be given *early* in the illness while the diagnosis is still only suspected and before the nature of the infection can be verified retrospectively by virological techniques, and before severity and localizing features justify brain biopsy.

This is something of a tall order, and general practitioners and physicians would need to be able to make this presumptive diagnosis early. But again I want to emphasize, as strongly as I can, that in this type of case it is always, I believe, a clinician's duty to be as sure as possible that the condition is not one of brain abscess or tuberculous meningitis. These themselves can be difficult enough diagnoses to make in the early stages, and ones that we still find are liable to be overlooked. These two diseases are today curable, whereas, whatever the future may hold for the treatment of herpes simplex encephalitis, there is as yet no specific remedy. Therefore, if there is any doubt *at all*, I am sure that one should act on the assumption that the case is one of abscess or tuberculous meningitis. To have to act in this sort of way is after all the everyday lot of the true empiric, whether or not he also regards himself as a scientist.

REFERENCES

MacCallum F.O., Potter J.M. & Edwards D.H. (1964). Early Diagnosis of Herpes Simplex Encephalitis by Brain Biopsy. *Lancet* ii, 332–334.

Herpes Simplex Encephalitis—Virological Diagnosis

A. H. Tomlinson & F. O. MacCallum

Since I was invited to discuss 'Virological Diagnosis' publications by Johnson *et al.* (1968) and by Miller & Ross (1968) have effectively covered the subject, but I will however, illustrate the virological problem from the results obtained on 10 patients* in the Radcliffe Infirmary between 1961–1967 under the care of Mr Pennybacker and Mr Potter.

The results in Table 2 illustrate the four patterns. First the ideal, with virus isolation and a 16-fold rise in antibody; patients L. R.,

TABLE 2. Summary of virological results on ten cases of herpes simplex encephalitis

| Patient | Virus Isolation | | | | Viral Antigen by FA | | Serum CF Titre+ | |
| | CSF | | Brain Biopsy | PM | | | | |
	Lumbar *	Ventr. *		*	Biopsy	PM ±	1st	2nd
L. R.			+				8	128
B. S.	0/1		+				<8	128
A. S.	0/3		+	0/4			16	256
W. P.	0/2		+	2/2	?	?	8	Died
R. L.	0/1	0/4	+	6/6		2/5	<8	Died
W. B.		0/2	+	8/13	+	8/13	64	Died
H. H.			−				8	32
K. H.							1000	64
R. A.	0/2		+				256	256
M. M.	0/1	1/1					64	128

A space in the table indicates that the test was not done.
* No. of specimens yielding virus/no. tested.
± No. of specimens showing specific fluorescence/no. tested.
+ Reciprocal of endpoint dilution.

B. S., A. S.; second, virus isolation and death before the rise in antibody titre, W. P., R. L., and W. B.; thirdly, diagnosis relying solely on the serology; patient H. H. showed a barely acceptable 4-fold rise and virus

*With the exception of W. B. all these cases have been described, or referred to, by MacCallum, Potter & Edwards (1964), or Buckley & MacCallum, (1967).

was not isolated. From patient K.H. the first serum (day 14) had a titre of 1 : 1000 which fell to 1 : 64 in two years. Fourthly diagnosis by virus isolation without significant change in titre; patient R.A. had fairly high unchanging titres and M.M. showed only a 2-fold rise. Grist (1967) studied a patient with an insignificant rise up to day 12, but the titre rose 8-fold by day 14, only 24 hours before death.

It is noteworthy that virus was not found in any of 10 specimens of lumbar CSF, and in only one of seven specimens of ventricular fluid, but was recovered from seven out of eight biopsy specimens.

There appear to be only three records of herpes simplex virus having been recovered from the CSF in cases of encephalitis (Gostling 1967, Hunt & Comer 1955, Brunell & Dodd 1964).

Tables 3 and 4 show the timing of the laboratory findings on two patients. The day on which clear signs of encephalitis presented is designated 'o'. Patient A.S. fell ill on day minus 3, on day plus 3 there were cells in the CSF but no detectable virus, although a biopsy taken on the same day yielded virus. On day 4, i.e. seven days after the probable start of symptoms, the antibody titre was 1 : 16, and it rose to 256, so this case appeared to be a primary infection. He died 15 months later and virus was not recovered at necropsy.

Patient W.B. had a history of herpes labialis, and an antibody titre of 1 : 64 on day 3; all consistent with persistent infection. On day 1 the CSF was unremarkable, on day 2 the biopsy tissue showed specific immunofluorescence and virus was grown in culture. He died on day 5.

TABLE 3. Synopsis of virological findings, patient A.S.

		CSF			
		Cells/		Biopsy	CFT
	Day	cu mm	Virus	Virus	Titre+
Headache, fever	−3				
onset, aphasia	o				
	3	310	−	+	
	4	440	−		16
	9	600	−		
	16				256
	180				256
Death	15 mos	No virus recovered at P.M.			

+ Reciprocal of endpoint dilution.
A space in the table indicates that the test was not done.

TABLE 4. Synopsis of virological findings. Patient W.B.

		CSF		Biopsy		
	Day	Cells/ cu mm	Virus	Virus	F.A.*	CFT Titre+
Dizziness	− 50					
Cold sore	− 7					
L. side weakness	− 1					
Onset, coma	0					
	1	4	N.D.			
	2			+	+	
	3					64
Death	5	Virus in 8/13 specimens at PM				

+ Reciprocal of endpoint dilution.
A space in the table indicates that the test was not done.
* F.A. fluorescent antibodies.

These cases expose two large gaps in our knowledge: (i) how long before onset (as defined above) does infection of the brain begin? A.S. was well until three days before onset whereas W.B. had complained of dizziness for six or seven weeks (ii) Why did A.S. who appeared to be a primary infection without antibody at the onset, survive, but W.B. who almost certainly had antibody before encephalitis, succumb rapidly?

Virus isolation
It is important to diagnose a case of herpes encephalitis quickly because of the possibility of using specific anti-viral therapy with iodo-deoxyuridine, the probable value of which will be discussed by Drs MacCallum and Mackenzie.

When a patient has a CNS infection with an enterovirus, or mumps, it is usually possible to isolate the virus from throat swab, faeces or cerebrospinal fluid, and the isolation of such a virus is always of some interest. In contrast, because latent infection with herpes virus is so wide-spread, the isolation of herpes virus from sites other than the brain, has little relevance to a diagnosis of encephalitis.

How early in the disease virus can be isolated turns therefore on how soon there are sufficient clinical indications to justify brain biopsy and even then, the neurological signs may be inadequate to localize the site of infection. No biopsy was done on patient M.M. for this reason (lack of localizing signs) but a sample of fluid removed during ventriculogram yielded virus.

Miller & Ross stated that in their series, virus isolation required two to seven days but we, culturing in primary human amnion cells, have had results more quickly. Of the eight specimens from which virus grew, seven showed a characteristic cytopathic effect in 42 hours, and the eighth was positive at 24 hours. As an indication of the value of amnion cells—a swab from herpes labialis has shown characteristic CPE in six hours—few virus isolations are more rapid.

Despite this ease of cultivation, some biopsy specimens produced only 1 to 10 foci of infection in the tubes, perhaps because of an element of chance in the sampling, or perhaps because the patient's antibody can interfere with viral growth.

Although I have emphasized the importance of biopsy in the search for herpes virus, the culture of throat swab, faeces and CSF for other neurotropic viruses must not be neglected.

Antibody levels

The assay of serum antibody is of little help in rapid diagnosis. A survey of the sera from 1029 people (Smith, Peutherer & MacCallum 1967) showed that at the age of one year, 15 to 20 % of children had detectable antibody to herpes simplex virus and the proportion rose to over 70 % by the fiftieth year. The estimation of viral antibodies is not well standardized between laboratories so it is not easy to compare absolute levels, but Smith *et al.* also quote figures for individuals with complement fixing titres of 1 : 32, a level which would be detected by any competent laboratory. Of 414 people aged 22 years and over, 50 % had titres of 1 : 32.

Leider *et al.* (1965) report the laboratory findings of 18 cases of encephalitis or meningitis attributed to herpes simplex virus, and Miller & Ross give details of 12 cases of encephalitis. In these 30 cases seven titres of 1 : 32 or higher were observed in the first five days of the disease, and 10 such titres in the first seven days. Antibody at this level could arise from previous infection, from recurrent herpes, or from the suspected brain infection and there is no way of distinguishing between them.

A 4-fold increase in antibody is generally accepted as significant and although this may occur within five days, more usually eight to ten days elapse, and so serology cannot provide a rapid diagnosis. There are reports of a rise of titre when a new vesicle appeared on patients with recurrent herpes and Johnson *et al.* suggest this as possible source of error in diagnosis. It is, however, generally believed that recurrences do not produce a rise in antibody (Dudgeon 1950, Holzel *et al.* 1953, Ross & Stevenson 1961).

The one occasion when a single serum sample may give suggestive evidence is when the first specimen available is taken late in the disease and has a titre in the region of 1 : 1000.

Hence if a patient with encephalitis shows a 4-fold or greater rise in herpes antibody, and no other aetiology is obvious, herpes simplex encephalitis is the most likely diagnosis, and the greater the increase in antibody the more probable is the diagnosis.

Identification of antigen with fluorescent antibody
Although immuno-fluorescence has been extensively tried as a diagnostic tool in microbiology—often with more enthusiasm than discrimination—it is a poor substitute for isolation of the virus or bacterium and when used in the search for one of several pathogens it is very laborious. However, in the search for a single pathogen and when speed is essential the technique is worth consideration. Because isolation of virus has usually taken two days we decided to do fluorescent staining whenever the biopsy specimen was large enough. I must emphasize that material for culture should have priority. A piece of tissue 1 × 2 mm was blocked in gelatin, frozen, sectioned in a cryostat, and several sections stained with test and control conjugates.

Although herpes antigen in mouse brain stained well, we experienced initial difficulties with human brain. These difficulties were overcome by careful control of non-specific staining and the use of serum from an intensively immunized rabbit.

Sections from the biopsy of patient L.P. gave an equivocal result, but those from W.B. showed 15 to 20 brightly fluorescent cells with no comparable fluorescence in the controls. No specific fluorescence was seen in biopsy material from six other patients who subsequently proved not to have herpes encephalitis. I am sure that fluorescent staining, applied with adequate controls and interpreted with care, is a useful aid to early diagnosis, but the chance of success depends very much on the extent of infection in the tissue sampled.

Fluorescent staining is, however, unique in its ability to show the disposition of infection in a post-mortem brain and is more informative than a search for inclusion bodies. Fluorescent cells were found in two lobes of R.L.'s. brain. Unfixed tissue was taken from 13 sites in

TABLE 5. Distribution of virus in brain of patient W. B. at death, five days after onset

	Left		Right	
	Virus isolation	Fluorescent cells*	Virus isolation	Fluorescent cells*
Frontal cortex	4+	5	−	50
Temporal cortex	4+	20	4+	100
Parietal cortex	4+	50	+	100
Occipital white matter	N.D.	N.D.	+	20
Occipital cortex	N.D.	N.D.	−	−
Central white matter	+	10	+	−
Cerebellum	−	−	−	−
Medulla	−	−	−	−

* Estimate of no. of cells stained by fluorescent antibody, in each low-power field.

the brain of W. B., for virus culture and fluorescent staining, which revealed many fluorescent cells, apparently neurones, in the cortex and very rare fluorescent small cells, possibly glial cells, in the white matter. Figures 5 to 8 illustrate the appearance of the sections. Table 5 summarizes a rough quantitation of the virus recovered and the number of fluorescent cells in different parts of the brain. The infection was widespread, despite treatment with iodo-deoxyuridine. The discrepancies between amounts of virus and numbers of fluorescent cells may be due to sampling, the imprecision of the technique or possibly, the more advanced necrosis in the right hemisphere allowed penetration of antibody and neutralization of virus.

Electron microscopy
Although electron microscopy has been fairly widely used to demonstrate herpes simplex virus in the postmortem brain of patients with encephalitis, the technique has been little used for rapid diagnosis on biopsy samples. Electron microscopy lacks the immunological specificity of immuno-fluorescence but it can demonstrate small numbers of particles which might not be associated with stainable antigen.

Conclusion
We conclude that isolation of virus from the brain appears to provide the only certain diagnosis, though isolation at necropsy can belatedly confirm a clinical diagnosis.

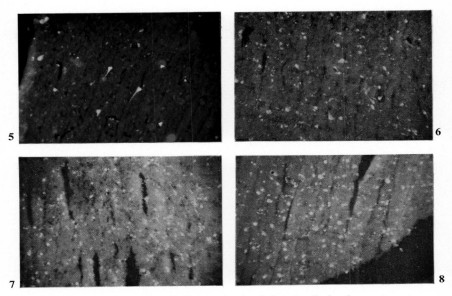

Immunofluorescent staining of Herpes simplex infected cells in the post-mortem brain of patient W. B.

FIGURE 5. Left temporal lobe
FIGURE 6. Left parietal lobe
FIGURE 7. Right temporal lobe
FIGURE 8. Right occipital lobe
Magnification: × 60.

When virus isolation is not possible, serological results, interpreted with care, may be a useful supplement to the clinical findings. It appears that a fair proportion of the cases reported in the literature have been diagnosed on very tenuous evidence, a fact already emphasized by Johnson *et al.*

REFERENCES

BRUNELL P.A. & DODD K. (1964) Isolation of *Herpesvirus hominum* from the cerebrospinal fluid of a child with bacterial meningitis and gingivostomatitis. *J. Pediat.* **65**, 53–56.

BUCKLEY T.F. & MACCALLUM F.O. (1967) Herpes simplex virus encephalitis treated with idoxuridine. *Brit. med. J.* ii, 419–420.

DUDGEON J.A. (1950) Complement fixation test for herpes simplex infections. *J. clin. Path.* **3**, 239–247.

GOSTLING J.V.T. (1967) Herpetic encephalitis *Proc. Roy. Soc. Med.* **60**, 693–696.

GRIST N.R. (1967) Acute viral infections of the nervous system. *Proc. Roy. Soc. Med.* **60**, 696–698.

HOLZEL A., FELDMAN G.V., TOBIN J.O'H. & Harper J. (1953) Herpes simplex: A study of complement fixing antibodies at different ages. *Acta paediat.* **42**, 206–214.

HUNT B.P. & COMER E.O'B., (1955) Herpetic meningo-encephalitis accompanying cutaneous herpes simplex. *Amer. J. Med.* **19**, 814–823.

JOHNSON R.T., OLSON L.C. & BUESCHER E.L. (1968) Herpes simplex virus infections of the nervous system. Problems in laboratory diagnosis. *Arch. Neurol. (Chicago)*, **18**, 260–264.

LEIDER W., MAGOFFIN R.L., LENNETTE E.H. & LEONARDS L.N.R. (1965) Herpes simplex virus encephalitis. *New Eng. J. Med.* **273**, 341–347.

MACCALLUM F.O., POTTER J.M. & EDWARDS D.H. (1964) Early diagnosis of herpes simplex encephalitis by brain biopsy. *Lancet*, ii, 332–334.

MILLER J.D. & ROSS C.A.C. (1968) Encephalitis: A four year survey. *Lancet*, i, 1121–1126.

ROSS C.A.C. & STEVENSON J. (1961) Herpes simplex meningoencephalitis. *Lancet*, ii, 682–685.

SMITH I.W., PEUTHERER J.R. & MACCALLUM F.O. (1967) The incidence of *Herpesvirus hominis* antibody in the population. *J. Hyg. Camb.* **65**, 395–408.

Pathology of Herpes Simplex Encephalitis

J. Trevor Hughes

The literature of this subject is extensive and I shall only cite four references. The first is a paper by Smith, Lennette & Reames (1941) which appeared in the *American Journal of Pathology* in 1941 and which reported the isolation of herpes simplex virus from the brain of a child who had died of encephalitis. This was probably the first acceptable report that cases of acute fatal encephalitis could be due to the herpes simplex virus. The other three papers I wish to mention are the paper of Haymaker (1949) in 1949, that of Dr van Bogaert and his colleagues (van Bogaert, Radermecker & Devos 1955) in 1955 and that of Krücke (1957) in 1957. Although there have been many reports since and a few that preceded these papers the recognition of a distinctive type of necrotic encephalitis with localization to one hemisphere, particularly the temporal lobe and nearby structures, was largely due to the careful descriptions in these three papers.

TABLE 6

Case no.	Sex	Age	Duration of illness	Virus grown (biopsy)	Virus grown (necropsy)	Virus seen (E.M.)
1 (W.P.)	M	43	3 days	+	+	
2 (R.L.)	M	18	4 days	+	+	+
3 (W.B.)	M	47	5 days	+	+	+
4 (D.O.)	F	73	16 days			+
5 (A.S.)	M	40	15 months	+	−	

My own remarks concern the findings at necropsy in five cases in which the association with herpes simplex virus was proven. Table 6 shows that in these five cases four had a positive virus isolation from a cerebral biopsy and from three of these virus was isolated at necropsy. Virus particles were demonstrated by electron microscopy on the necropsy tissue of three cases.

I have arranged these five cases according to the interval that elapsed from the onset of the severe neurological illness to death. In this way a

29

study of cases 1 to 3 showed the pathological picture in the first few days of the illness, the fourth case with death at 16 days shows a more established degree of cerebral inflammation whilst the last case shows the appearance in the brain after a survival period of 15 months.

In my lecture, I dealt with the localization of the disease by showing numerous colour slides of the brain specimens. In this published account the localization and the degree of brain necrosis, as judged by histological examination, is given in Table 7. It is apparent that although in all five cases bilateral encephalitic changes were present there was always a greater involvement of one cerebral hemisphere. Also certain cortical areas such as the insula, gyrus rectus, superior middle and inferior temporal gyri, hippocampal gyrus, occipito-temporal gyrus, and cingulate gyrus were always involved to a greater degree than any other cortical areas. The localization to these areas of the severe encephalitis is of great interest and has provoked much speculation. I wish to direct attention to the remarkable attack of the virus on the limbic lobe and the limbic system. From the medial aspect of one cerebral hemisphere the cingulate gyrus, the isthmus, the hippocampal gyrus, and the uncus appear in the form of a ring of cerebral cortex which is sometimes called the limbic lobe. The term limbic system refers to the limbic lobe together with certain connecting tracts and associated internal nuclei. The neuronal structure of the cortex throughout the limbic lobe is similar and so we have the possibility of a special susceptibility to an attacking virus. I much prefer the idea of an anatomical pathway of infection along the olfactory nerve to the gyrus rectus and so to both the cingulate gyrus and the hippocampus. We have not found gross changes in the olfactory nerve but the virus may pass this way without causing a severe local effect.

Whilst the preferential involvement of the limbic lobe of one cerebral hemisphere is such a feature of this disease, it must be emphasized that there is also widespread involvement of the remainder of the brain. Table 7 shows that microscopical evidence of encephalitis was present in regions as remote as the pons. The recovery of the virus from the brain *post mortem* (Table 8) also gave evidence of the widespread distribution, always bilateral, of the herpes simplex virus and its greater concentration in the cortical areas already mentioned.

We now come to consider the histological changes in this disease. Fig. 9 depicts a myelin-stained section from a coronal slice of the left hemisphere. This is case 2 with death at four days and we see here the early pathological picture. Note the severe oedema which in the cortex

TABLE 7. Distribution of encephalitic lesions

	Case 1 (W.P.)		Case 2 (R.L.)		Case 3 (W.B.)		Case 4 (D.O.)		Case 5 (A.S.)	
	left	right	left	right	left	right	left	right	left	right
Superior frontal gyrus	—	+	+	—	—	+	+	—	+	—
Middle frontal gyrus	—	++	+	+	—	+	++	+	+	—
Inferior frontal gyrus	+	++	+	+	+	++	+++	++	+++	++
Insula	++	+++	+++	+	++	+++	+++	+++	+++	++
Orbital gyri	+	++	++	+	+	++	+++	+	++	+
Gyrus rectus	+	+++	+	+	+	+	++	+	++	+
Gyri of parietal lobe	—	+	+	—	—	+	+	—	+	—
Gyri of occipital lobe	—	+	+	—	—	+	+	—	+	—
Superior temporal gyrus	+	+++	+++	+	+	+++	+++	+++	+++	++
Middle temporal gyrus	+	+++	+++	+	+	+++	+++	+++	+++	++
Inferior temporal gyrus	+	+++	+++	+	+	+++	+++	+++	+++	++
Hippocampal gyrus	++	+++	+++	+	+	+++	+++	+++	+++	++
Occipito-temporal gyrus	++	+++	++	+	+	++	+++	+++	+++	++
Cingulate gyrus	++	+++	++	+	+	+++	++	+	+++	++
Midbrain	++		++		++		++		+	
Pons	+		+		+		+		—	
Medulla	—		—		—		—		—	
Cerebellum	—		—		—		—		—	
Spinal cord	—		—						—	

+ + + Confluent areas of necrosis.
+ Microscopical changes

+ + Non-confluent foci of necrosis.
— No encephalitic changes.

J.Trevor Hughes

TABLE 3. Recovery of virus at necropsy

	Case 1 (W.P.)		Case 2 (R.L.)		Case 3 (W.B.)		Case 5 (A.S.)	
	Left	Right	Left	Right	Left	Right	Left	Right
Frontal lobe		−	+	±	−	+ +	−	
Temporal lobe	+	+	+ +	+	+ +	+ +	−	−
Parietal lobe		−	±	±	±	+ +		
Brain stem							−	
Cerebellum					−	−		

gives the vesicular appearance and picks out the involved cortex of the temporal lobe, the insula and the cingulate gyrus. Figure 10 depicts the detail of this oedematous cortex. This low power photomicrograph shows the round oedematous areas in the centre of which (Fig. 11) are dying neurone cell bodies surrounded by clusters of microglia. This phenomenon of degenerating neurones surrounded by microglia is called neuronophagia. The inflammatory exudate is mainly of lymphocytes and monocytic phagocytes with very few polymorphonuclear leucocytes. Even in an area of intense cortical destruction (Fig. 12) there are few polymorphs although because of the break up of nuclei into smaller nuclear fragments an extensive polymorph exudate may be wrongly identified. The break up of the nuclei is the effect of the virus particle within the nucleus and to see this we should at this point examine the ultrastructure of the nuclei (Figs. 13a and b). We have looked for and found virus particles in three out of three of these cases. They are easy to find because of this vacuolar degeneration of the nucleus with the condensation of the chromatin material into these smaller electron-dense portions. With practice these nuclear changes can be seen at quite low magnification and this allows one to pick out the nuclei containing virus particles. The virus particles are about 1000 Å in diameter and have the shape of a dough-nut (Fig 13b) but sometimes with a central core.

Returning to the light microscopical picture, I will comment on the cerebral vessels in this disease. An effect frequently seen in the vessel wall is that the endothelium is swollen and abnormally permeable. Sometimes one can see a small vessel such as a capillary blocked by recent thrombus. These thrombotic changes may explain the intense

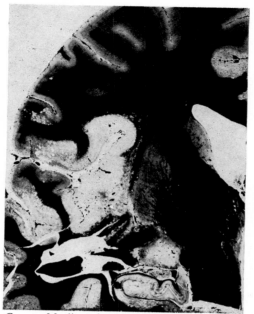

FIGURE 9. *Case* 2. Myelin-stained celloidin section of the left cerebral hemisphere cut coronally at the level of the thalamus. Note the oedema in the temporal lobe, in the insula, and in the cingulate gyrus. (Kulschitsky-Pal. × 1½.)

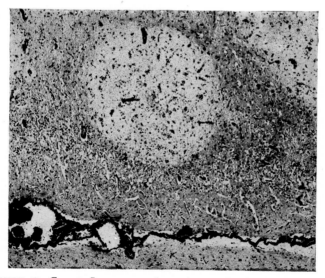

FIGURE 10. *Case* 2. Low-power photomicrograph of the cortex of the temporal lobe, showing several round oedematous areas of necrosis. (Haematoxylin and eosin, × 50).

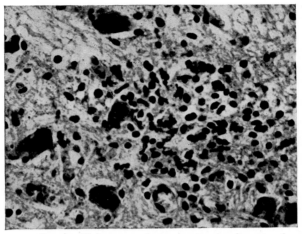

FIGURE 11. *Case* 2. High-power photomicrograph of neuronal necrosis and neuronophagia. (Haematoxylin and eosin, × 250).

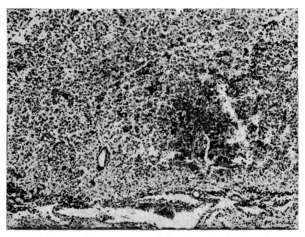

FIGURE 12. *Case* 4. Low-power photomicrograph showing confluent necrosis of the cortex of the temporal lobe. (Haematoxylin and eosin, × 50).

FIGURE 13. *Case* 3. Electron micrographs of formalin-fixed cerebral white matter post-fixed in O_sO_4. From araldite-embedded blocks, ultra-thin sections were cut and stained with 2 % aqueous uranyl acetate and lead citrate. (a) Nucleus of ? oligodendroglial cell undergoing vacuolar degeneration and fragmentation into smaller electron-dense nuclear masses. (× 21,200). (b) Detail of virus particle present in Figure 13a (× 63,000).

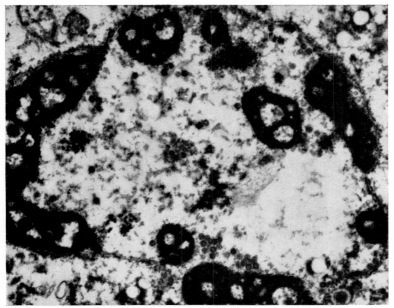

(a)

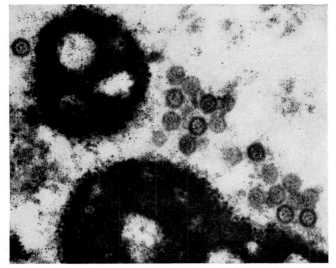

(b)

necrosis which gives an appearance very similar to infarction. In the case with survival to 16 days, the whole cerebral cortex was necrotic (Fig. 12) and the amount of tissue damage was as great as that seen in infarction caused by vessel occlusion. The inflammatory cells seen in these cases are either small lymphocytes or monocytic phagocytes. Very characteristic is a perivascular cuffing (Fig. 14) with lymphocytes which in Fig. 14 are seen around a small penetrating cortical vessel.

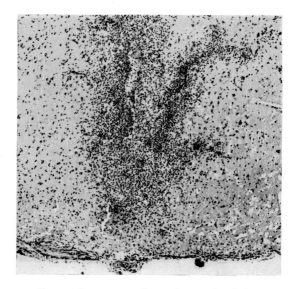

FIGURE 14. *Case* 1. Low-power photomicrograph of the cortex of the temporal lobe showing perivascular cuffing of small penetrating cortical vessels. (Haematoxylin and eosin, × 50).

The end result of the attack of encephalitis was seen in case 5 with survival to 15 months. Figure 15 shows a section from the left cerebral hemisphere with extensive damage to the insula, the temporal lobe and to the cingulate gyrus. In the damaged areas the cortex has been completely destroyed and there remains only a rim of subpial tissue forming the wall of a cyst cavity.

This ends my survey of the acute and long term pathological picture in herpes simplex encephalitis. I hope that this account will stimulate discussion of the puzzling features of this interesting disease.

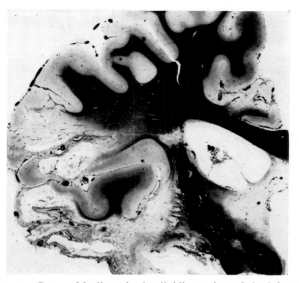

FIGURE 15. *Case* 5. Myelin-stained celloidin section of the left cerebral hemisphere cut coronally at the level of the thalamus. Note the cystic cavities caused by the former necrosis (15 months earlier) in the temporal lobe, in the insula, and in the cingulate gyrus. (Kulschitsky-Pal. × 1½).

REFERENCES

HAYMAKER W. (1949). Herpes simplex encephalitis in man, with report of 3 cases. *J. Neuropath. & Exp. Neurol.* **8**, 132–154.

KRÜCKE W. (1957). Über eine besondere Form der spontanen Encephalitis. *Nervenarzt.* **28**, 289–301.

SMITH M.G., LENNETTE E.H. & REAMES H.R. (1941). Isolation of virus of herpes simplex and demonstration of intranuclear inclusions in case of acute encephalitis. *Amer. J. Path.* **17**, 55–68.

VAN BOGAERT L., RADERMECKER J. and DEVOS J. (1955). Sur une observation mortelle d'encéphalitis aigue necrosante. *Rev. neurol.* **92**, 329–356.

Herpes Simplex Virus Encephalitis: summing up

F. O. MacCallum

You have heard from my colleagues of the manner in which the cases seen here have presented themselves and the steps which we, like others, have taken to improve the speed of diagnosis. It is my task to discuss briefly these findings and other available information on the pathogenesis of the disease, particularly in relation to the possibility of achieving benefit to the patient by specific treatment, which was one of the main aims of the urge to obtain a more rapid diagnosis.

This is not a very common disease as far as is known at present, but it is probably one of the commonest single causes of sporadic severe virus encephalitis, other than that associated with chickenpox or measles, in this country. In the United Oxford Hospitals in the past seven years there have been seven adults and one 11-year-old child from whose brain (7) or ventricle fluid (1) the virus was recovered and two other adults in whom the pathology and/or serology supported the diagnosis. Only the child made a complete recovery. Dr Hughes has also mentioned a few other patients in whom postmortem brain was shown to have pathological lesions suggestive of HSV infection but in whom no virological studies were made. During the same period of seven years there was only one patient resident in the area admitted with paralytic poliomyelitis and one, possibly two, patients with subacute sclerosing panencephalitis admitted to the hospital from other areas.

Two other examples of the prevalence of HSV encephalitis in Great Britain in recent years were the 12 cases occurring during the period 1964–1967 in the Institute of Neurological Sciences in Glasgow, recently reported by Miller & Ross (1968) and four cases from the Portsmouth area in 1966 reported by Gostling (1967). In passing, it is of interest that in Glasgow in 1966 (Grist 1967) only one of 221 patients with aseptic meningitis had a rising titre of antibody to HSV and this was an infant. We have not encountered a rise in antibody to HSV in 200 to 300 cases of aseptic meningitis in the past seven years.

It may be that there are a number of patients in mental institutions or at home whose mental disability of varying degree is due to herpes simplex virus in the past, but no technique is available for determining this unless the brain is available postmortem and even this may not be helpful.

It has been recognized for many years that the majority of primary infections with herpes simplex occur in infancy and early childhood as stomatitis or gingivo-stomatitis which is frequently unrecognized but primary infection may also occur in adults. It tends to be a family infection. If mother has it she also has antibodies which pass through the placenta and protect the infant for the first three to six months. After this the infant becomes susceptible and is infected by older siblings or parents. Although the majority of primary infections occur in childhood in large sections of the population in whom attack rates of 70 to 90% are found, in other groups, such as medical students and nurses and those from a higher socio-economic level only 30 to 50% have been infected by the twenty-fifth year. Once infection has occurred the virus remains in the body for the remainder of the patient's life as do the antibodies in the blood.

Viraemia may occur, probably in only a small proportion of patients, at the time of the primary infection at any age. Although the virus has a predilection for tissues derived from the embryonic ectoderm it may also involve mesodermal tissues as is seen in disseminated herpes of the new born or of young children with Kwashiorkor or severe measles in Africa. When disseminated herpes occurs in the new born, encephalitis is often present. Most recorded cases have been fatal but survival with mental retardation has been described. A less severe or unrecognized infection in which the virus as a result of viraemia lodges and remains latent in the brain or other organs such as the liver, may occur in an unknown number of patients.

After the description of the first fatal cases of HSV encephalitis in adults in the 1940's and later when interest in this disease increased, I think that it was generally believed that these were primary infections. Certainly none of the early cases investigated here had a history of herpetic infection and virus was found in the nose or throat in only one. As Dr Tomlinson has mentioned, the last patient investigated in the Radcliffe Infirmary in December 1967, W.B., was the only one out of the ten investigated here to date who had a past history of recurrent cold sores. Some of the first few patients with a very rapid progressive onset had no antibody in their acute serum and others with a more delayed course had a low titre of antibody on admission but had an increase in titre if they survived a week or more. However, in 1965,

Leider and his colleagues in San Francisco reported three cases of encephalitis in adults who had a history of recurrent labial herpes and acceptable rises in titre of complement-fixing antibody: virus was isolated from the brain of one of these patients postmortem. These latter observations taken together with earlier experiments which showed reactivation of HSV encephalitis in previously infected rabbits by the production of anaphylaxis or by peripheral injection of adrenaline led to the hypothesis by Leider *et al.* and others that some cases of HSV encephalitis are the result of a reactivation of a long-standing infection in the brain while others are primary infections. The mechanism of latent infection with HSV anywhere in the body is still a mystery. The genome of the virus may become incorporated in certain susceptible cells in which little or no complete virus is produced, thus enabling the ability to replicate to persist and the virus to be reactivated when suitable conditions are provided. It is possible that neutralizing antibody and interferon usually prevents spread outside the cell, but in tissue cultures virus has been shown to spread to contiguous cells in the presence of antibody and produce either no visible change or microscopic changes in the infected cells. It is also possible that naked virus DNA can escape from cells in an infective form and this will not be neutralized by antibody. In addition to spread by viraemia the virus may spread along nerves in the endoneural cells and might travel from the nose to the brain along the olfactory nerves. Although numerous strains of herpes produce encephalitis in rabbits after corneal inoculation I have not found any record of a case where this was suspected in man, and there have been only a few reports where CNS involvement has followed skin lesions at different sites as in the experimental disease in animals.

As has been mentioned already, although most of these patients with encephalitis have signs of a meningitis, virus has been reported isolated from lumbar CSF of only two adults—and one of these also had Boeck's sarcoid and other unusual features (Hunt & Comer 1955)—and from the ventricular fluid of one patient here whose lumbar fluid was negative (Buckley & MacCallum 1967). The results of investigations of one acute case (W.P.) and the last two patients seen here who had been ill at least 10 days when admitted (M.M., R.A.) indicated that inability to recover virus from the CSF was not due to the presence of antibody in it. The latter patients survived some months with severe cerebral deficit in other hospitals and a small number of specimens of CSF were obtained at intervals. The blood was positive at high titre but no virus or antibody was present in the CSF at the time of admission to hospital. Antibody appeared within seven to ten days and gradually increased until the titre was only about 2-fold less than that of the blood. A high titre persisted in the CSF for at least three months in one (M. M.) but had fallen to a low level after five months in the other (R. A.). Although no conclusions can be drawn from the results on only three patients the blood/CSF ratio in the early convalescent period in the two patients who survived was much lower than that seen for measles antibody in patients with subacute sclerosing panencephalitis (Connolly *et al.* 1967).

The only other report I have found of virus infection of the CNS in which the titres were similar in the CSF and blood in a proportion of patients, is that of Dr Webb and his colleagues who studied the therapeutic effect of an avirulent strain of tickborne encephalitis virus in patients with leukaemia or neoplastic disease (Webb *et al.* 1966).

In addition to these points, evidence has been accumulating in the past few years that HSV, once thought to be a single immunological type in man, probably consists of two or more groups and some of our diagnostic virology has not caught up with this yet. Numerous strains of virus isolated from genital lesions have been only partly neutralized by antibody prepared against strains from recurrent skin lesions. Neonatal infections may be from either type. All the serological tests for identification of HSV infection in the past have been based on viruses from skin or brain so that the diagnosis may have been missed in some patients where only serological tests were done and negative or in some cases where acute necrotizing encephalitis was present, no virus was isolated and serology was negative, although in our limited experience there appears to be a common CF antigen and antibody between the two groups as seen in infected humans.

Also the molecular weight of the virus and its structure indicate that the virus DNA can code for about 50 proteins and Wildy and his colleagues and others have already found evidence of at least 12 antigens by immunodiffusion tests so that identification of virus antigen as incomplete or non-infectious virus by immunofluorescence will depend to a high degree upon the virus preparation used to prepare the antiserum used in the test.

Thus we are presented with three possible situations for treatment.
1   Acute fulminating encephalitis in an infant, usually as part of a disseminated infection. This is a primary infection and considered to have a very high mortality rate.

2   Acute fulminating encephalitis in older children, adolescents and adults. A primary infection with no antibody in the serum. There is a high mortality rate and a cerebral deficit in a high proportion of those who survive. Children under 15 are considered to have a better prognosis than adults.

3   Acute encephalitis, sometimes with symptoms of a preceding history of illness suggestive of low-grade brain disease for a week or more. Antibody is present in the blood on admission and sometimes there is a history of recurrent herpetic lesions of the skin. The prognosis is poor.

Dr Mackenzie is going to discuss treatment of virus disease in the CNS in general, but I shall consider specific treatment with 5-iodo 2-deoxyuridine (IDU) in herpes encephalitis. As you know, this drug, which is an analogue of thymidine, interferes with replication of HSV, which is a DNA virus. This has been shown in tissue culture and also in acute infection of rabbit and human cornea and in guinea-pig skin and in recurrent lesions in human skin if treatment commences early enough with a high concentration of the drug.   However, although there is macroscopic evidence of more rapid healing of the lesions in these various sites the virus is not necessarily eliminated.

What chance have we then of interfering with replication and spread of the virus in the brain by the use of this drug? It is potentially toxic, attacking the DNA of dividing cells, thus, fortunately, not normal neurones. It has a low solubility in neutral solutions; it is broken down into inactive components within about four hours *in vivo*; it is relatively unstable on storage, retaining its activity only two to three weeks at the pH required to keep it in solution at the optimum concentration, 0·5%, which is five times stronger than the stock preparations for use in the eye. This means the solution must be prepared freshly as soon as the diagnosis is made.

The basis for considering the use of this drug in HSV encephalitis and the dose to be used were the reported experience of systemic use of the drug in man for treatment of patients with malignant disease in the period 1960–1965 by Welch, Prusoff, Calabresi and their colleagues at Yale. Delayed toxicity in the form of alopecia, leucopaenia, and stomatitis occurred in a small proportion of their patients given the maximum total dose of 600 mg/kg intravenously over five days. Dr Mackenzie will be discussing experimental results of Tokumaru in HSV encephalitis in guinea-pigs. It is perhaps of passing interest that the decision to treat the first patient in the USA and in this country occurred at approximately the same time in 1965. Because of doubts concerning the toxicity of the drug Mr Pennybacker's patient, who did not have clearly defined localizing signs, was treated with a relatively small dose through a canula in the carotid artery on one side for five days. There was no change in the patient's clinical condition which could be attributed to the drug (Buckley & MacCallum 1967). In Boston the now well-known adult patient of Breeden, Paul & Tyler (1966) was treated with decompression followed by a total dose of 600 mg/kg of IDU intravenously over five days. The patient, who had been in a coma for several days when treatment commenced, made an extremely good recovery, although he was left with a partial visual defect—(his wife thought he was normal!)—but as the authors pointed out recovery is known to occur in a small proportion of patients who have not received IDU. Thus the drug appeared to be worth a further trial. In the case of the 13-year-old boy treated by Marshall (1967) marked improvement occurred within 36 hours of decompression and commencement of intravenous IDU. It is difficult to attribute this rapid reaction to the action of the drug although it may have helped in recovery. We have not found any further published reports, but the last patient seen here, W.B. (already mentioned by Dr Tomlinson), who had had only a few days history of acute CNS disease, died after 48 hours of intravenous treatment with the maximum dosage and as you saw virus was recovered from numerous sites in the brain obtained postmortem.

There is no available information on what proportion of the drug given intravenously reaches the brain substance in an affected brain and ideally I suppose that intraventricular inoculation should also be given. As is so often the case in medicine, the patients whom the drug may appear to benefit most are those with the best chance of survival without treatment. However, until some more efficient drug is found it seems worthwhile to continue to use IDU with an unbiased approach and great efforts should be made to attempt to monitor its action on the brain and on the virus in all possible ways. A controlled trial is obviously not possible. Thus in conclusion the question I put to you is whether one should continue to use the drug or not!

REFERENCES

Breeden C.J., Hall T.C. & Tyler R.H. (1966) Herpes simplex encephalitis treated with systemic 5-iodo-2′-deoxyuridine. *Ann. Intern. Med.* **65**, 1050–1056.
Buckley T.F. & MacCallum F.O. (1967) Herpes simplex virus encephalitis treated with idoxuridine. *Brit. med. J.* ii, 419–420.

CONNOLLY J.H., ALLEN I., HURWITZ L.J. & MILLAR J.D. (1967) Measles virus antibody and antigen in subacute sclerosing panencephalitis. *Lancet* i, 542–544.
HUNT B.P. & COMER E. (1955) Herpetic meningo-encephalitis accompanying cutaneous herpes simplex. *Amer. J. Med.* **19**, 814–823.
GOSTLING J.V.T. (1967) Herpetic encephalitis. *Proc. roy. Soc. Med.* **60**, 693–702.
GRIST N.R. (1967) Personal communication.
LEIDER W., MAGOFFIN R.L., LENNETTE E.H. & LEONARDS L.N.R. (1965) Herpes simplex virus encephalitis. *New Engl. J. Med.* **273**, 341–347.
MILLER J.D. & ROSS C.A.C. (1968) Encephalitis: A four year survey. *Lancet*, i, 1121–1126.
WEBB H.E., WETHERLEY-MEIN G., SMITH C.E.G. & MCMAHON D. (1966) Leukaemia and neoplastic processes treated with Langat and Kyasanur Forest disease viruses: a clinical and laboratory study of 28 patients. *Brit. med. J.* i, 258–266.

The Problem of Acute Encephalopathy in Children

By B. D. Bower

The main problem for the paediatrician is the separation and identification of the treatable conditions which present as acute encephalopathy from those which are untreatable. Until very recently viral encephalitis was in the latter group, but with the emergence of a treatment for herpes simplex encephalitis, it may be moving into the group of treatable conditions and the precise diagnosis of acute encephalopathy is becoming more urgent.

Acute viral encephalitis is a great mimicker and diagnosis is notoriously difficult. A history of head injury, for instance, is commonly obtained, especially in the young toddler, and such a history makes it imperative to consider the possibility of intracranial haemorrhage of one sort or another. The following case of Coxsackie B encephalitis is an example of this, and also forms a reasonably good—one cannot use the word 'typical'—example of acute viral encephalitis:

This was a boy aged five years who was quite well until he fell when out shopping with his mother and bruised his left temple. He was not concussed. Five days later he seemed quieter than usual and it was noticed that his speech was slightly slurred, he was drooling from one side of his mouth, and his gait was slightly unsteady. His family doctor found one extensor plantar response and he was admitted to the Radcliffe Infirmary into the Accident Service (Mr J. Potter) ten days after the fall. At that time examination showed him to be a little slow in carrying out commands and he had a mild right hemiparesis. Investigations showed: a mid-line echo on the echoencephalogram, a normal left carotid arteriogram, an EEG with marked bilateral slow wave activity with some high-voltage, stereotyped, slow-wave complexes rather reminiscent of subacute sclerosing leuco-encephalopathy (however, these were not seen on any of the subsequent 11 weekly records), and CSF containing 16 cells/cu mm (15 lymphocytes) with normal chemistry.

From this point there was a rapid deterioration in his conscious level with increasing spastic quadriplegia and the onset of major, focal, and myoclonic fits. He was discharged home after four months, virtually a spastic, quadriplegic ament. A brain biopsy had shown shrunken and pyknotic cortical cells, with a doubtful increase in small glial cells and several small vessels cuffed with cells that look like phagocytes . . . 'The appearance is compatible with encephalitis, but no positive diagnosis can be made on this alone' (Dr D. Oppenheimer). Coxsackie B2 virus was isolated from fluid from each lateral ventricle and from his stools.

Here an acute virus encephalitis was eventually proved, but the rapid exclusion of other causes of acute encephalopathy was needed.

I shall now discuss some other conditions which encephalitis may mimic in childhood and mention some aids to diagnosis, in the main to the diagnosis of conditions *other than* encephalitis. Diagnosis by exclusion is unsatisfactory. There is a great need, made more urgent by the fact that specific anti-viral therapy may be just round the corner, for *rapid* reliable laboratory aids to a positive diagnosis.

Acute encephalopathy is hardly a precise entity but we need waste no time trying to define it. Two almost constant clinical features are *interference with conscious level* and *convulsions*, and a variety of neurological signs and symptoms may accompany these two. In considering acute rather than subacute encephalopathy, we should define the onset in hours or days, rather than weeks. The *first* condition which springs to the paediatrician's mind is *pyogenic meningo-encephalitis*, because it is the easiest to treat and because treatment is urgent; the ultimate result in terms of intelligence closely depends upon the time which elapses before antibiotics are started. Diagnosis is easy once CSF is available, unless antibiotics have masked the typical CSF picture, and I shall say no more about this condition; nor about *cerebral abscess or tumour*, conditions which are notoriously easy to *mis*diagnose but about which much has been written. A good example of the difficulty in diagnosis is that of a child of 14 months with only a five day history of illness and 24 hour history of fits. She was drowsy on admission with a mild unilateral upper motor neurone lesion. CSF contained 82 cells (66% lymphocytes) and normal chemistry. She had a glioblastoma multiforme. Interestingly, her lumbar CSF and rectal swab grew a Coxsackie B2 virus, which was prevalent in the Oxford area at the time. Nor shall I discuss tuberculous meningitis, a notorious diagnostic trap, for Dr Honor Smith is to consider this in her contribution.

When convulsions are a prominent feature of the presentation, the encephalopathy has rather different aetiological implications. The child, previously quite well or with a minor infection, suddenly starts to convulse and rapidly goes into status epilepticus. This may be the result of virus encephalitis, but is often not. Status epilepticus can itself so interfere with cerebral function that encephalitis is simulated, and it is difficult to know whether the continuance of the epileptic state is alone responsible for the coma and neurological signs, or whether the encephalopathy is the result of encephalitis.

When fits are unilateral and a hemiplegia occurs the terms 'acute infantile hemiplegia', 'acute hemiplegia of childhood' or 'hemiplegia, hemiconvulsions and epilepsy' (Gastaut *et al.* 1957) have been used. This syndrome has intrigued many since Freud first described it in 1897 and it was clear in the early descriptions that there are several causes. Middle cerebral artery thrombosis, venous sinus thrombosis, and encephalitis have each been found in the relatively few cases who come to autopsy. Encephalitis has always seemed a rare cause, for the CSF is usually normal, although I doubt if many cases have been examined by modern virological techniques. Bickerstaff's important paper (1964) showed that middle cerebral artery occlusion was a frequent cause of the syndrome. He demonstrated that carotid arteriography in the acute phase would in most cases show a filling defect in the middle cerebral artery territory and often also in the carotid at tonsillar level, and suggested spread of infection from an acute tonsillitis to the adjacent internal carotid artery. Carotid arteriography in the acute phase is now indicated, for anticoagulant therapy has to be considered.

Acute encephalopathy may be iatrogenic, following immunization, usually from the pertussis antigen. Diagnosis should not be difficult when symptoms follow rapidly but may be more difficult when the latent period between immunization and the onset of symptoms is longer. The syndrome of infantile spasms with mental regression is one form of encephalopathy which may follow closely upon immunization and I have seen about 30 patients over the years in whom I have felt that the encephalopathy was caused by immunization. Unfortunately there is no means of proving it.

Another encephalopathic syndrome in which convulsions are a dramatic feature is Reye's syndrome, or the wet brain—fatty liver syndrome. Reye and his colleagues described in 1963 a condition in which an infant or young child suddenly starts to vomit and within one to three days becomes comatose with convulsions. The liver enlarges in the first few days and hyperpnoea is common. The most frequent biochemical abnormalities are hypoglycaemia and raised serum transaminases. Metabolic acidosis is common. At autopsy fatty degeneration of liver and kidneys and cerebral oedema are present. The condition presents problems. Is the encephalopathy secondary to hypoglycaemia which in some patients may be transient and therefore missed; or are the brain and liver both affected by some as yet unidentified toxic substance? Is there an inborn error of metabolism in these children which causes a normally harmless dose of, for instance, salicylates to be profoundly toxic to both brain and liver?

Certain poisons also have to be considered, and in children between one and four years lead is a notorious mimic of encephalitis. In Britain today the patient is likely to be an immigrant living in an old house with layers of old paint on the woodwork, the deeper layers containing lead. The child may chew the paint out of sheer boredom. One day he starts to convulse and is admitted to hospital convulsing and comatose with signs of raised intracranial pressure. Because of language difficulties the history of pica and of some previous vomiting or abdominal pain may not be obtained. The CSF usually shows a raised protein, which may suggest a cerebral tumour. If the condition is thought of, an X-ray of the wrist to show the dense lead line at the metaphyses and of the abdomen to show the flakes of lead paint in the bowel, should give the correct diagnosis.

Iron salts are also not infrequently swallowed by exploratory toddlers. An unexplained coma with convulsions can be due to this cause, though here a history of ingestion of ferrous sulphate tablets is usually available. Other poisons in young children can cause more bizarre encephalopathies. Atropine (in eye ointments or as deadly nightshade berries) causes acute mania and then coma and convulsions. Amphetamine presents a similar picture. Imipramine causes stupor, convulsions, and attacks of opisthotonos and choreo-athetoid movements. An important feature in such cases is the common occurrence of a variety of cardiac arrhythmias. Barbiturates and antihistamines, of course, produce stupor and ataxia followed by coma without such dramatic features.

So far I have been considering encephalopathy affecting predominantly the cerebrum. But in young children particularly, an acute *cerebellar* encephalopathy may occur. The child develops over a day or two gross ataxia of gait and stance, with intention tremor of the arms and nystagmus, often gross, oscillatory, and non-lateralized. Intracranial pressure is usually normal and the CSF is either normal or contains a slight excess of cells. It is important to distinguish this from a cerebellar tumour for the prognosis is nearly always good and craniotomy obviously unnecessary. The aetiology is various: true virus infection, for instance poliomyelitis, chickenpox, measles, ECHO and influenza, has been found in some cases; others have followed vaccination with polio and triple vaccine. Even a closed head injury has produced it.

I have tried to show that a wide variety of agents can cause acute encephalopathy in childhood and that the clinician must be aware of this. He must ask the right questions in history-taking and then initiate the appropriate investigations.

REFERENCES

BICKERSTAFF E. R. (1964) Aetiology of acute hemiplegia in childhood. *Brit. Med. J.* ii, 82–87.

GASTAUT H., VIGOROUX M. TREVISAN C. & REGIS H. (1957) Hemiplegie, hemiconvulsion, epilepsie (Syndrome H.H.E.) *Rev. Neurol.* **97**, 37–40.

REYE R. D. K., MORGAN G. & BARAL J. (1963) Encephalopathy and fatty degeneration of viscera in childhood. *Lancet* ii, 749–752.

CSF Findings in differential Diagnosis

H. V. Smith

Mr Potter has pointed out that the confusion between viral infections of the central nervous system and tuberculous meningitis or brain abscess is not only easy but may be disastrous. It seemed worthwhile, therefore, to see if any clues to differential diagnosis could be obtained from examination of cell counts and the protein content in cerebrospinal fluid (CSF).

There are 35 estimations from 27 proven cases of tuberculous meningitis chosen at random from the Oxford series. I have also collected 35 estimations from 27 proven cases of brain abscess from the records of the Neurosurgical Department. Finally there are 24 estimations from presumed or proven cases of viral infections collected from the records of the United Oxford Hospitals. The cases of proven herpes encephalitis already discussed are included: the findings in these cases are distinguished in the graphs but their distribution does not, in fact, differ from those of the group as a whole. All estimations were made before any intrathecal injections were given and before any intracranial operation. They are, therefore, unaffected by such changes in cell count or protein content as may follow these procedures.

The findings are summarized in four simple histograms (Figs. 16–19) which form unsophisticated distribution curves. In all the figures the findings for tuberculous meningitis are at the top, the viral infections in the middle and the abscesses at the bottom. Since the numbers are small, absolute figures are given but the percentage formed by each sub-group of one group as a whole, is marked at the head of each column.

First, the distribution of lymphocytes and polymorphonuclear leucocytes: there is a traditional view that a preponderance of polymorphs will occur with abscesses and that the presence of these cells almost excludes tuberculous meningitis. Figure 16 shows the percentage of lymphocytes in the three conditions we are considering. The central dotted line represents 50%. In all, over 70% show a preponderance of lymphocytes.

Comparison of the total cell counts is more informative (Fig. 17).

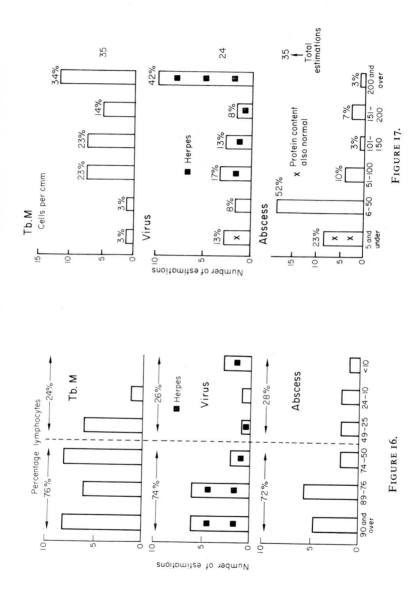

FIGURE 16.

FIGURE 17.

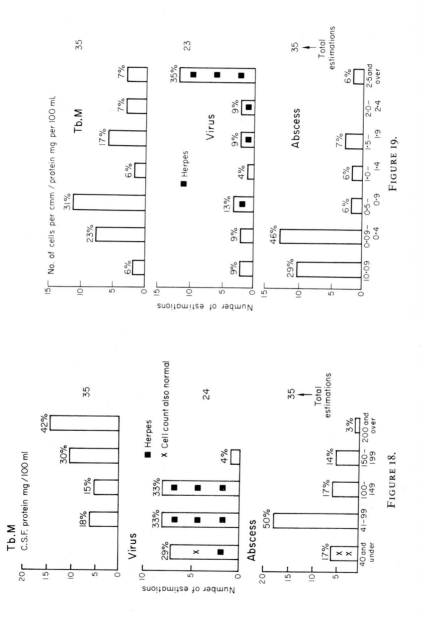

FIGURE 19.

FIGURE 18.

Estimations are recorded in units of 50 along the abscissae. The normal range is of five cells per cu mm and under. In three of the viral estimations falling in the normal range, and in three also of the abscess estimations, but in none of the tuberculous ones, the protein content was also normal, that is the fluids were normal in all respects. Otherwise both the tuberculous and the viral fluids show a fair number of cells; indeed the two curves follow one another quite closely with the viral counts, in particular, peaking sharply at 200 per cu mm and over. By contrast, the abscess counts peak equally sharply at between six and 50 cells per cu mm, that is at the other end of the scale.

Figure 18 shows the protein content. Here the differences appear to run in the opposite direction. The tuberculous cases produce more protein than either of the other two groups. The abscesses once again peak fairly sharply at the 41–99 mg of protein level. Only six had a normal protein. The viruses distribute themselves equally amongst the lower ranges but a protein of over 150 is exceptional. Thus in 70% of the tuberculous fluids the protein was above 150 mg per 100 ml while only 4% of the viruses and 17% of the abscesses fall there.

It seems, therefore, that both the viral infections and the tuberculous infections tend to produce more cells than do the abscesses. The abscess fluids, on the other hand, may contain rather more protein (17% above 150 mg per 100 ml) than the viral. A rise in protein is the rule in the tuberculous cases. This difference can be highlighted by dividing the number of cells by the amount of protein in mg per 100 ml and expressing the result as a simple ratio.

Figure 19 illustrates this. The difference between the abscesses and the viruses is well shown, with the former tending to peak in the lower ratios (0·4 and under) and the latter in the higher (2·5 and over). Figures for tuberculous meningitis simply reflect the well-known tendency for the protein rise to follow the cell count in this condition so that ratios tend to peak about unity. However, even though 70% of abscesses show ratios of below 0·4 and 50% of viruses show ratios of 1·5 and higher, nevertheless there is still an overlap and the differential diagnosis is still not beyond doubt.

These figures can show where the probabilities of diagnosis lie. However, it is important to remember the small overlap, and to realize that in no given case can the possibility of either abscess or tuberculous meningitis be ruled out by examination of the CSF.

Acute Encephalopathy in Children

D. R. Oppenheimer

Some cases of acute encephalopathy, after presenting a diagnostic problem to the paediatricians, die and present a diagnostic problem to the neuropathologists. About 1400 necropsies are performed each year at the Radcliffe Infirmary, of which about 40 are on infants aged between one month and five years, dying of all causes. Of these 40, one or two have died as a result of the condition I am going to talk about. In our post-mortem material on this age group, it is one of the commonest neurological causes of death—commoner, for instance, than all the strictly inflammatory diseases of the brain or meninges put together.

A typical case history runs like this. A three-year-old child is unwell for a week or so, with a mild upper respiratory complaint. One day he vomits, becomes drowsy, then unconscious, and proceeds to have major convulsions. The temperature rises to 40°C or over. The lumbar fluid contains a normal amount of protein, and less than 5 cells per cu mm. Virological studies of blood and CSF are normal. The neurological state deteriorates, and the child dies within about a week from cardiac or respiratory arrest. The clinical diagnosis is usually of acute (?viral) encephalitis.

At necropsy, the brain is generally swollen, sometimes to the point of herniation through the tentorial incisura, causing brainstem compression. Histologically, there is cerebral oedema, and widespread changes in nerve cells characteristic of cerebral anoxia. There is no sign of inflammation. No virus is recovered from the cerebral tissue. The liver is enlarged and fatty, and the lungs show a not very severe pneumonia, of a type suggestive of a virus infection. The other viscera are unremarkable.

This is a composite picture, based on 15 cases examined here during the past 10 years. They are all in children, only one of whom was over four years of age. Among the variants of this pattern, a few deserve special mention. Firstly, at least two of the cases had had previous fits—either in the form of so-called febrile convulsions or as grand mal epilepsy. In both these, the brains showed damage due to earlier convulsions. Secondly, the acute illness was preceded, in several cases, by specific viral infections. Two had had measles within the previous two weeks; one had been vaccinated against smallpox one week before; one had varicella two months before; and one, at the time of her illness, had a very high titre of antibodies to the respiratory syncytial virus. In one case, showing the histology of a severe virus pneumonia, adenovirus 7 was isolated from lung tissue after death. In no case was the herpes simplex virus implicated, and in none was there shown to be a specific bacterial infection. Biochemical disturbances, including raised blood urea and impaired liver function, were noted in several cases. In one, there was a blood sugar below 20 mg%. The period between the onset of the acute illness and death varied between one and 17 days, with a mean of three days.

Turning to the pathology of the brain, the changes have always been widespread and non-specific, but of varying severity. In the first place, there is generalized cerebral oedema. Secondly, there are the common so-called anoxic changes—shrunken nuclei and eosinophilic cytoplasm—which may result from a variety of disturbances, including circulatory arrest, hypoglycaemia and status epilepticus. Equally common is an appearance which seems to be due to waterlogging of the cytoplasm of nerve cells and neuroglia, and which is rarely seen in adult brains but is relatively common in those of acutely sick children. The cerebral cortex is usually affected in one or both of these ways, and in two cases, in which the illness had lasted a week or more, there was frank cortical infarction. The cerebral white matter shows oedema of varying severity; but in no case has there been any sign of the perivenous tissue destruction characteristic of post-exanthematous or post-vaccinal encephalitis.

In the viscera, only the lungs and the liver have shown significant changes. About half the cases had a bronchopneumonia at the time of death, which did not seem to be due to bacterial infection. The liver in most cases was swollen and fatty—a not uncommon finding in acutely sick children; but in a few cases there were more specific lesions, such as inflammatory cell infiltration (one case) and areas of focal necrosis (three cases). Unfortunately, the livers from these cases with definite signs of hepatitis were not examined virologically.

Whatever part these pulmonary and hepatic lesions play in the course of the disease, the dominant clinical features are clearly the result of cerebral damage. When we ask what mechanisms might produce this damage, we are faced with a long list of theoretical possibilities:

1   *Virus in brain*. This cannot be ruled out, in spite of consistent failure

to isolate virus. Absence of histological signs of inflammation is not conclusive evidence against it.

2 *Circulating toxins.* These have always been the principal suspects. In none of our cases was there any evidence implicating pathogenic bacteria; thus one has to think in terms of toxins released by tissues infected by virus, or possibly of liver damage, with failure to detoxicate substances originating in the gut.

3 *Exogenous poisons.* Here we have no positive evidence; but one has to bear in mind the possibility of abnormal reactions to therapeutic drugs given during the prodromal phase.

4 *Allergy.* The classical post-infective perivenous encephalitis is histologically indistinguishable from the experimental so-called allergic encephalitis which can be produced in animals by injections of brain tissue with adjuvant. The condition which we are discussing is histologically very different from this—and incidentally appears to be a much commoner complication of vaccination, measles, and other infections. It is possible that it represents an alternative 'allergic' reaction on the part of the brain; but I do not know of any report of its having been induced in experimental animals.

5 *Hypoglycaemia.* This has been observed in a minority of reported cases. When it occurs, it is probably attributable to liver damage. Brain cells, especially in the cerebral cortex, are known to be susceptible to severe or protracted hypoglycaemia.

6 *Epilepsy.* The fits, which occur in nearly every case, are presumably the result of some sort of damage to nervous tissue; on the other hand, severe and protracted fits produce a characteristic pattern of damage to the juvenile brain, and it is certain that many of the grosser lesions we observe are the result, and not the cause, of the epilepsy.

7 *Hypoxia.* Again, the observed 'hypoxic' changes in nerve cells are commonly seen after status epilepticus, and their occurrence in these cases cannot be definitely ascribed to one cause or another.

8 *Cerebral oedema.* This, too, is a frequent concomitant of cerebral hypoxia and of status epilepticus. When severe, it results in herniation, and is the immediate cause of death.

9 *Chemical imbalance.* Dehydration, and disturbances of pH and electrolyte balance, undoubtedly occur in many cases; but what part these play in the cerebral pathology is at present quite obscure.

10 *Hyperpyrexia.* This is said to cause damage, especially to the cerebellum; but the high fever in these cases generally occurs several hours *after* the onset of fits and the development of coma.

The picture emerging from these rather confusing bits of evidence appears to be something like this. There is an acute cerebral illness, often associated with virus infections, but never shown to be due to the presence of virus in the brain. It is commonly fatal in infants, but rarely in older children or adults. The clinical picture in fulminating cases is fairly characteristic, but it is almost impossible to decide how often the same condition occurs in a milder form, with complete or partial recovery, or whether these fatal cases, with their high fever, coma and epileptic fits form a continuum with the apparently harmless 'febrile convulsions' of infancy. The clinical diagnosis is nearly always 'acute (?virus) encephalitis', whereas the usual post-mortem diagnosis is 'acute "toxic" encephalopathy'. I suspect that this verbal discrepancy may have some psychological importance. As things are at present, a diagnosis of virus encephalitis is apt to engender an attitude of fatalism, whereas the suspicion of a biochemical disturbance is a stimulus to investigate the case as fully as possible, and to attempt to correct whatever imbalance is discovered.

A very detailed, but inconclusive, discussion of the problem of aetiology, by a group of Boston clinicians and pathologists, appeared in 1961 (Lyon, Dodge & Adams 1961), and there have been several papers since then stressing the frequency of liver damage and of hypoglycaemia in cases of this kind. Since rational treatment depends on knowledge of causal mechanisms, and since it is probable that there are multiple causes at work in individual cases, there is clearly need for research on several different lines; but of all these the most important, I think, is the investigation of the nature of these shadowy 'toxic substances' which are released into the body fluids in the course of certain virus infections, and the effects of these substances on immature nervous tissue.

REFERENCES

LYON G., DODGE P.R. & ADAMS R.D. (1961): The acute encephalopathies of obscure origin in infants and children. *Brain*, **84**, 680–708.

Aspects of Diagnosis

E. M. Brett

Loss or impairment of consciousness, with or without convulsions, is the most dramatic manifestation of encephalitis in children, and these features are not peculiar to the cerebral disorder of encephalitis, but may occur in a wide variety of other conditions affecting children. The nervous system of the child may be acutely affected by a wider range of baneful influences than operates in later life, and the young nervous system seems to have a limited repertoire of reaction, so that the clinical picture produced by different agents may be very similar.

The history is very important, but this may present difficulties of interpretation in the child.

Thus, there is sometimes uncertainty, especially with infants, about the patient's pre-morbid normality or abnormality. This will depend on a detailed developmental and perinatal history, which may not be available.

In childhood, especially in the schoolchild, infections of all kinds, bacterial, viral and of uncertain origin are common. In most childhood illness enquiry will disclose a history of a recent upper respiratory infection of banal type, or of a specific infectious fever, and the significance of this in relation to a neurological syndrome is often difficult to assess. Local knowledge of what neurotropic virus diseases are occurring in the community at the time may be valuable, although it can also at times be misleading. A history of infection may suggest encephalitis and divert attention from the true diagnosis, as in the case of brain-stem or cerebellar neoplasms presenting soon after an attack of measles or chicken-pox.

Trauma is almost universal in a paediatric history, and its significance is, therefore, also difficult to assess. Traumatic subdural haematoma must be included in the differential diagnosis of encephalitis. The index of suspicion for trauma must be high, since injury may be denied, and bruising, fractures or retinal haemorrhages may bear witness to it in the case of the 'battered baby syndrome'.

In any childhood illness, poisoning with toxic substances must be considered, since it is an increasingly common cause of coma with or without seizures, as has been mentioned by Dr Bower.

Drugs may be taken by a child accidentally, a term which includes the feeding of a toddler by an older child with a parental medication. It is perhaps almost as common for a child to be poisoned by being given an overdose of a drug or drugs prescribed for him. Overdosage with hydantoin in this way is a common cause of severe ataxia and an occasional cause of coma in children. Measurement of the blood level of barbiturate or hydantoin may be needed in doubtful cases.

Specific side-effects of certain drugs may give rise to suspicion of encephalitis. These include the dramatic dyskinesias, trismus and psychic disturbances sometimes seen in children taking phenothiazine drugs (Cottom & Newman 1966). Raised intracranial pressure may occur in children treated with tetracycline and nalidixic acid, and also during the course of treatment with adrenocortical steroids and ACTH while the dose is being reduced.

Biochemical disturbances in children may simulate encephalitic illnesses. Hypoglycaemia and hypo- or hypercalcaemia may be associated with convulsions and altered consciousness, and the blood levels of sugar, calcium and electrolytes should be measured in all children presenting with impairment of consciousness so that appropriate treatment may begin as soon as possible. Chemical disorders occurring in the course of acute dehydrating illness in children, either as a result of vomiting or diarrhoea, or of treatment, may lead to severe neurological complications of such illnesses, which may be wrongly attributed to encephalitis. Hypernatraemic dehydration in infants resulting from injudicious use of salt in the feeds is often associated with brain damage, and carries a particular risk of convulsions during the stage of rehydration. Seizures may result from water-intoxication in the treatment of dehydration. The combination of fever and dehydration in some infants is followed by thrombosis of the superior longitudinal sinus and its branches with neurological sequelae which may be labelled 'encephalitic', since the appropriate radiological tests are rarely made.

Immunizing procedures in infancy carry an appreciable risk of adverse reactions. This is particularly true of triple vaccination with DPT in which the pertussis element seems to be the neurotoxic factor. A recent Swedish study (Ström 1967) showed an incidence of neurological reactions of 1 in 3600 vaccinated children. Amongst other neurological syndromes, provocation of hypsarrhythmia was seen in four cases, as previously suspected by American and British workers (Baird & Borofsky 1957, Bower & Jeavons 1960) and there were three cases of 'severe cerebral injury', two of which showed decerebrate rigidity.

Several infants have recently been seen at the Hospital for Sick Children, Great Ormond Street, in which a severe encephalopathic illness has followed a triple vaccination. The calamity has followed the second or third injection, rather than the first, as was commoner in the Swedish series. The encephalopathic illnesses following DPT are sometimes attributed to viral encephalitis, but viral studies rarely support this view.

Convulsions in childhood often present a problem for the paediatrician in deciding the relationship between the seizures and the rest of the clinical picture; whether acute neurological and mental deterioration is secondary to the fits, whether fits and deterioration are both secondary to a single cerebral pathology, such as encephalitis, or to a biochemical disorder, or whether both situations may obtain. 'Acute infantile hemiplegia' or acute hemiplegia in childhood as Dr Bower mentioned, illustrates this difficulty. Prolonged 'febrile convulsions' in infants are sometimes followed by lasting neurological deficit, and when this happens the evidence of the fever-provoking infection, usually upper respiratory, leads often to a diagnosis of viral encephalitis. In most such cases, this is not justified by the results of CSF, viral and other investigations, and has the harmful effect of diverting attention from the urgent need to control status epilepticus, of which so-called febrile convulsions are the commonest 'cause' in infancy. The role of status epilepticus and febrile convulsions in the aetiology of temporal lobe epilepsy has been argued convincingly by Ounsted and his colleagues (1966).

Four case histories of children with acute encephalopathic illnesses may be mentioned briefly to illustrate some of the diagnostic difficulties. One case concerned a boy of seven with an acute 'toxic' encephalopathy and slow recovery. Another involved a two year old girl who became severely demented with rigidity following prolonged status epilepticus with a febrile coryza. CSF and viral studies were negative in both these cases, and there seemed no justification for a diagnosis of viral encephalitis. By contrast a five month old boy who developed a hemiparesis and blindness following fever and fits showed an increase in CSF cells and protein, and viral studies suggested a recent Coxsackie B2 infection, so that viral encephalitis seemed likely. Rubella encephalitis was strongly suggested by the clinical, CSF and viral findings in a five year old girl whose illness occurred in a community where rubella was known to be prevalent.

E. M. Brett

REFERENCES

BAIRD H.W. & BOROFSKY L.G. (1957) Infantile myoclonic seizures. *J. Pediat.* **50,** 332–339.

BOWER B.D. & JEAVONS P.M. (1960) Complications of immunization. *Brit. med. J.* ii, 1453.

COTTOM D.G. & NEWMAN C.G.H. (1966) Dystonic reactions to phenothiazine derivatives. *Arch. Dis. Childh.* **41,** 551–553.

OUNSTED C., LINDSAY J. & NORMAN R. (1966) *Biological Factors in Temporal Lobe Epilepsy. Clinics in Developmental Medicine No.* 22. London.

STRÖM J. (1967) Further experiences of reactions to triple vaccination. *Brit. med. J.* iv, 320.

Aspects of Treatment

A. M. R. Mackenzie

The requirements of a specific chemotherapeutic agent directed against a virus are more difficult to meet than are the requirements of an anti-bacterial chemotherapeutic agent. Dr MacCallum described the use of idoxuridine (IDU) in the treatment of herpes simplex encephalitis. This agent is active in the treatment of cold sores and herpetic keratitis. The systemic toxicity of IDU prevents its use other than as a topical agent or in desperate situations, and its physical properties leave much to be desired. There are other compounds which have been shown to have *in vivo* anti-virus activity, but IDU is the only one which has so far been used in CNS disease. IDU appears to act by competitive inhibition of thymidine, an essential component of DNA (Eidinoff, Cheong & Rick 1959).

There has been, in the last four years, much discussion about the therapeutic potentialities of interferon (Finter 1968). This is a term including many polypeptides which inhibit virus multiplication. It is a problem to transport such substances to the site where they are required to act, and it would be particularly difficult to ensure that an interferon molecule penetrated to a neurone. Endogenously produced interferon is probably important in recovery from virus infections and from the therapeutic point of view it may be that agents actively inducing the formation of endogenous interferon will prove of more value than administration of the preformed compound. At the moment, however, particularly in the context of the present discussion, interferon has found no great therapeutic application.

Administration of γ-globulin during the incubation period of measles attenuates or aborts the attack. There is evidence that γ-globulin given in this way prevents the onset of encephalitis, but it does not appear to have any effect on the outcome if it is administered after the onset of encephalitic symptoms (Greenburg *et al.* 1955). There is evidence, discussed elsewhere in this symposium, that antibodies may have a deleterious effect in encephalitis and with this in mind it might be considered on first principles to be unwise to give γ-globulin for acute encephalitis.

The use of steroids in virus infections is a complex subject, about which much has been written. There is laboratory evidence that steroids *in vitro* enhance rather than inhibit virus replication (Kilbourne & Horsfall 1951). In addition interferon synthesis and action are suppressed (Kilbourne, Smart & Pokorny 1961). In many experiments with living animals the picture is the same. It was found many years ago that cortisone exacerbates the effect of poliovirus in monkeys (Sabin & Fieldsteel 1952). It has also been shown in hamsters that the pathological processes accompanying poliovirus infection are enhanced by cortisone administration and that poliovirus causes paralysis when inoculated intraperitoneally into an animal treated with steroids whereas in an animal not treated with steroids virus given by this route does not lead to paralysis (Schwartzman 1954). Intradermal vaccinia in rabbits usually gives rise to local skin lesions, but rabbits treated with steroids develop a rapidly fatal generalized infection (Bugbee, Stewart & Like 1958, Campillo-Sainz *et al.* 1961).

In the clinical situation vaccination is generally acknowledged to be a dangerous procedure in patients on steroids. The local application of steroids to some patients with zoster and herpes simplex results in severe exacerbation of the lesions and silent latent infection may be unmasked in this way. However, these examples represent situations in which the primary pathology is cell destruction due to virus replication and it would probably be undesirable to suppress an antigen-antibody reaction. In certain forms of encephalitis there is evidence that inflammatory changes and undesirable antigen-antibody reactions may contribute more to the eventual damage than virus replication and in these situations the administration of steroids may be desirable. Most of the clinical literature on this topic is concerned with measles encephalitis and reports on the value of steroids in this condition are conflicting (Appelbaum & Abler 1956, Allen 1957, Meade 1959, Karelitz & Eisenberg 1961, Ziegra 1961, Katz 1962, Boughton 1964). Some of this confusion may result from a failure to differentiate between acute meningo-encephalitis accompanying measles and post-infectious encephalitis.

An experimental situation similar to human herpes simplex encephalitis has been described recently (Tokumaru 1968). Guinea-pigs were inoculated intracerebrally with herpes simplex virus, various treatments were given and the effect of these on the survival rate and mean survival time was measured. IDU and interferon each had a therapeutic effect when administered as a five day course. Inoculation of a fraction of purified guinea-pig globulin was effective up to 60 hours after infection. At this time exponential multiplication of virus began, and by 72 hours globulin was ineffective. Hydrocortisone had no therapeutic effect at all, given either as a single dose or a five day course.

In these experiments the brains of the guinea-pigs were infected suddenly by a large dose of virus, a situation which probably does not arise in human herpes simplex encephalitis. These results cannot therefore be considered without reservation to be entirely applicable to man.

In summary, chemotherapy for encephalitis shows promise, interferon may find future application when technical difficulties are overcome, and the value of steroids is still controversial.

REFERENCES

ALLEN J. E. (1957) Treatment of measles encephalitis with adrenal steroids. *Pediatrics* (*NY*), **20**, 87–91.

APPELBAUM E. & ABLER C. (1956) Treatment of measles encephalitis with corticotropin. *Am. J. Dis. Child.* **92**, 147–151.

BOUGHTON C. R. (1964) Morbilli in Sydney: A review of 3601 cases with consideration of morbidity, mortality and measles encephalitis. *Med. J. Aust.* ii, 859–865. Morbilli in Sydney II: Neurological sequelae of morbilli. *Med. J. Aust.* ii, 908–915.

BUGBEE L. M., STEWART R. B., & LIKE A. A. (1958) The effects of cortisone acetate on intradermally induced vaccinia infection in rabbits. *Am. J. Dis. Child.* **96**, 608.

CAMPILLO-SAINZ C., SALIDO-RENGELL F. & GAMA M. A. (1961) Effect of topical application of hydrocortisone on dermic lesions produced in rabbits by vaccinia virus. *Proc. Soc. exp. Biol. Med.* **108**, 67–70.

EIDINOFF M. L., CHEONG L. & RICK M. A. (1959) Incorporation of unnatural pyrimidine bases into deoxyribonucleic acid of mammalian cells. *Science*, **129**, 1550–1551.

FINTER N. B. (1968) Of mice and men: Studies with interferon in Ciba Symposium on Interferon 204–217.

GREENBURG M., APPELBAUM E., PELLITTERI O. & EISENSTEIN D. T. (1955) Measles encephalitis I. Prophylactic effect of gamma globulin. *J. Pediat.* **46**, 642–647.

KARELITZ S. & EISENBERG M. (1961) Measles encephalitis. Evaluation of treatment with adrenocorticotropin and adrenal corticosteroids. *Pediatrics* (*NY*), **27**, 811–818.

KATZ S. L. (1962) Measles—its complications, treatment and prophylaxis. *Med. Clin. N. Amer.* **46**, 1163–1175.

KILBOURNE E. D. & HORSFALL F. L. (1951) Increased virus in eggs injected with cortisone. *Proc. Soc. exp. Biol. Med.* **76**, 116–118.

KILBOURNE E. D., SMART K. M. & POKORNY B. A. (1961) Inhibition by cortisone of the synthesis and action of interferon. *Nature* (*Lond.*) **190**, 650–651.

MEADE R.H. (1959) Common viral infections in childhood: a discussion of measles, German measles, mumps, chickenpox, vaccinia and smallpox. *Med. Clin. N. Amer.* **43**, 1355–1377.

SABIN A.B. & FIELDSTEEL A.H. (1952) Effect of certain hormones and other chemical compounds on experimental poliomyelitis. *Amer. J. Dis. Child.* **84**, 464.

SHWARTZMAN G. (1954) New aspects of pathogenesis of experimental poliomyelitis *Journal of Mount Sinai Hospital, New York*, **21**, 3–18.

TOKUMARU T. (1968) The protective effect of different immunoglobulins against herpes encephalitis and skin infection in guinea pigs. *Arch. für die ges. Virusforsch.* **22**, 332–348.

ZIEGRA S.R. (1961) Corticosteroid treatment for measles encephalitis. *J. Pediat.* **59**, 322–323.

Discussion

CHAIRMAN [MacCALLUM]: From various comments I think it would be best first to give an opportunity for questions to Dr Tyrrell.

WEBB: I am interested in the ability of viruses to transform cells and I would like Dr Tyrrell to try and tell me what part of a virus, or is it something that is produced by the virus cycle, may produce this transformation. Does it have to be a nucleic acid or could it be some other substance. The arboviruses are now well incriminated as causing transformation and I suspect many more will soon be shown to do so.

TYRRELL: I think it would be best if Professor Waterson and I answered this together. It depends really what you mean by transformation. You can change the composition of a cell when it becomes parasitized so that the virus multiplies, the cell produces antigens and if you stain it with fluorescent antibody you show that the antigens are there. Yet in a tissue culture system and probably sometimes in the intact host, the virus is alive, the cell is alive and thus things remain. But if you use transformation in the technical sense, used by tumour virologists, I think you should get your answer from Professor Waterson.

WATERSON: That has been put admirably by Dr Tyrrell. I shall be speaking a little later and won't steal my own thunder now.

SPILLANE: The neurologist, if not the virologist is beginning to appreciate the mysteries and complexities of this subject. I had hoped that earlier this morning we might have had more time for questions because the clinical phenomena are known to us but the interpretation is quite bewildering. You were describing the anatomy and physiology of the virus, but when a clinician sees a child with chickenpox or an old man of 70 dying of herpes simplex encephalitis, what is the clue to the activity of this virus; why in one case should chickenpox produce a rash in a child and in another case produce a fatal encephalitis? Why can you sometimes find the virus in CSF and sometimes not? Why do you find the virus in the living brain at times, and in autopsy you can't confirm that what you found was the virus? Is replication, which seems vital to produce what we call a disease, the property only of the nucleic acid?

TYRRELL: I must apologize for not explaining everything, but I think we can bridge some of these gaps on the basis of the principles I gave you earlier. For instance why does varicella zoster virus produce chickenpox in a child and fatal encephalitis in an old man? Primarily because the zoster virus is a virus which has a tropism, a tendency to multiply in cells of epithelial origin, either nervous cells or epithelial cells. You can show this in the laboratory. We have been doing work on this in organ cultures and if you put a virus, like a rhinovirus on top of cartilage or bone nothing happens; the virus does not multiply in these cells. Now we do not understand why this is but if you put it on epithelial cells it does multiply. So this tropism of the zoster virus for epithelial or neuronal cells explains why it goes to those cells rather than to the liver or to subcutaneous tissues. Why does it do one in one case and one in another? This is probably related to the way in which the virus enters the body and initiates infection. In the case of the child with chickenpox this child had no antibody; it inhaled the virus; the virus began to multiply somewhere on the mucous surfaces of the respiratory tract; it then spread into the bloodstream; circulated through the blood; found there, as it was trapped in a capillary somewhere, adjacent epithelial cells; it liked these; it multiplied in them and there may well have been an immune reaction between a little bit of antibody produced in the epithelium, and then the rash occurred. But some of the virus in the old man when he got chickenpox as a child may have remained in the cells of the nervous system somewhere, possibly in posterior horn cells, and then over the period of time represented by perhaps 60 years, antibody titres died down and the virus began to multiply again, maybe causing an ophthalmic herpes or something like that. The virus is the same but in a host with some immunity in which the virus starts multiplying again from a nerve cell, the clinical picture is quite different and it may spread out towards the skin or to the cornea or in through the nervous system to cause an encephalitis. This is the sort of way in which we can re-interpret the clinical data in terms of what we know now about how viruses multiply.

You asked a question about virus recovery. Basically there is one fact you have got to remember about nearly all viruses, they are very unstable. If you sneeze out viruses they die off extremely fast; if you put them on a swab and take them to the laboratory the swab dries out, particularly if it is warm, and the virus will all be gone by the time you get there. The same thing, in fact, happens in tissues. Very shortly, within a matter of hours at the latest, probably minutes in many cases, after the cells have died—remember the viruses are utterly dependent on cells—no more virus multiplication takes place in the dead cell and what virus was there disappears. So if you want to recover influenza virus from a case of influenzal pneumonia you have got to do the post-mortem within an hour or so of death. You have got to chill the body immediately after death occurs and, in addition, when a virus is inside the living cell it is protected from antibody. Immediately death occurs, membranes become permeable, antibody can get into the cell, into tissue spaces probably, and it can inactivate virus from which it has been separated by the cell membrane. So both thermal inactivation and neutralization go on very rapidly after death and this is probably the reason why you get no virus recoveries. Dr MacCallum gets them from biopsies and cannot get them with exactly the same techniques from dead tissue even very shortly after death.

WHITTY: Firstly Dr Tyrrell, is there any evidence that the viruses enter *damaged* cells more easily; and secondly is there any evidence that the behaviour of the replicate differs in any recognizable way from the original particle?

TYRRELL: The first question was about damaged cells. It's quite clear that the physiological state of a cell does influence the way the virus behaves when it gets into it. This is obvious when you think of how the virus replicates, using cell ribosomes and so on. I won't give many generalizations, but going back to my question of organ cultures and my pet rhinoviruses, we know that cells which are differentiated and producing mucus and metabolizing are extremely susceptible to rhinoviruses. Cells deeper in the same layer, the basal cell of the same epithelium, do not support the growth of the virus: those very cells which, if allowed to differentiate would in fact behave like the susceptible cells. Now when we are talking about trauma I think we may be talking about two different things. There is no doubt clinically that if you scratched the conjunctiva of a human being you could make it susceptible to adenovirus which would not grow on the intact conjunctiva. The two different things which may occur, I think, are first that the truly susceptible cells are made accessible because the surface epithelium has been destroyed. This may be the reason why wart virus infects when scratched, and vaccinia virus infects when a child scratches it into another area, and why we can get a vaccinia virus to take by pricking through, though not by just laying on, the epithelium. The other thing is that the very damaged cells, because of their physiological state are in fact more susceptible. This has been shown experimentally with polio virus. If you scarify the skin the cells which are healing, the fibroblasts, which are multiplying, will in fact be susceptible to virus infection whereas the skin in its healthy state where the fibroblasts are dormant will not be. Trauma may work in both ways. Going back to polio again, there is the earlier work of Dr Ritchie Russell and others, which showed that neurones which have been exercised are more susceptible to damage by polio virus. Whether this means that the virus multiplies better or whether it means that when multiplication occurs the cell is more likely to be damaged, one doesn't know. Certainly trauma, physiological as well as mechanical, can influence susceptibility to virus infections.

Your second question, is the replicate different in any way? Well, it can be. Where you have got a virus like a myxovirus which, in fact, uses some of the cell components to form the particle surface, if you take a virus from say a chick, it is going to have chicken protein in it. If you then make that virus infect a human cell you will get a virus out, which has got human protein in it. So it may be different. In general, however, the whole point about the virus is that it specifies from its own genetic information the unique properties of the material required for the finished particle.

MacCallum: What about receptors?

Tyrrell: I mentioned in a diagram that the virus sticks to the surface of the cell and then enters it. This is telescoping a great deal of information. Electrostatic forces are often responsible, in a general way, for the virus attaching, but whether these forces operate or not depends on the exact nature of the surface of the virus and the surface of the cell. Some viruses will attach only to certain cells.

But beyond that there does seem evidence that certain ingredients in the cell surface, receptors as Dr MacCallum said, allow the virus to come into a special contact with the cell so that it can be broken open and infection can be initiated. In the case of polio there are certain lipo-proteins present and a chicken cell, for instance, has not got the lipo-proteins which are present in the human cells so you cannot put a polio virus on it and infect it. The interesting thing is that if you take the polio virus and nucleic acid out of its coat and force it into the cell by some laboratory trick, the polio virus will then multiply inside a chicken cell. Part of the reason for this differential susceptibility probably lies in whether or not there are the right sort of receptors in the right part of the cell, so that the initial stage of virus multiplication can get underway.

PALLIS: I would like to ask Dr Tomlinson a question on the laboratory diagnosis of these viral infections. The clinician is always taught that to make a satisfactory laboratory diagnosis you have got to show the 4-fold increase in antibody titre, show Cowdry type A intra-nuclear inclusions and, if possible, isolate or culture the virus. Now my question relates to the 4-fold increase in antibody titre. I can understand that this is a relevant criterion for infections like arbo-virus or echo virus or coxsackie virus, and so on where the virus is not continuously in the body. But when the virus is continuously in the body like the herpes simplex virus and where we know it can flare up from some completely non-specific kind of provocation, how relevant is the 4-fold increase in titre? Could it be that a patient just has a febrile disease, maybe an encephalitis or not, and shows a 4-fold increase in antibody titre which has really got nothing to do with his neurological illness? One of your cases (case H.H. on your first chart) had as the only diagnostic criterion for calling it a case of herpes simplex encephalitis, a 4-fold increase. My second question is a clinical point. I have found it helpful in diagnosis of herpes simplex encephalitis that in many cases you find red cells in the spinal fluid in the very first lumbar puncture. These tend to be disregarded as traumatic. But in a patient who goes gradually into coma, if a lumbar puncture is done within the first 12 hours and shows red cells and even more xanthochromia, in my experience this has nearly always turned out to be a case of herpes simplex encephalitis.

TOMLINSON: To answer the point about antibody rises, I think I mentioned, but not very clearly, that when a patient with a recurrent herpes gets a new vesicle the general body of evidence is that he does not get a rise in antibody titre. A paper by Dudgeon in 1950, a survey in the middle fifties by Holzel and other people, and Ross & Stephenson in a paper about 1961, all mention this. Dr MacCallum has looked at quite a lot of recurrent herpetics here—some hundreds —without observing any rise in antibody on recurrence of ordinary herpes labialis. In the paper by Johnson and co-workers it is suggested that there may occasionally be a rise and this is a possible confusion. On the whole the evidence seems to be against this. It may possibly occur in the first one or two reactivations after the primary infection. Primary infection gives you a primary response of antibody which can climb—maybe in the first one or two recurrences there would be an increase in antibody—but the literature on the whole discounts an increase in antibody from many recurrences.

PALLIS: But S or V antibody?

TOMLINSON: Well measured by complement fixation or by neutralization. We may get more light on this in the future. The question about cerebrospinal fluid changes is, I think, one for Dr Honor Smith.

SMITH: When I was going through these fluids I did in every case list the red cells. I did not notice any obvious difference between the groups and, of course, small traumatic bleeds are common in anyone who has had a lumbar puncture whatever is wrong with him. One important point is that the blood, whether it is traumatic or not, is a most potent cause of artifact in the spinal fluid. Counts of 8000 to 10,000 red cells will really invalidate the white cell count and the protein content and for several days.

WELLS: May I first make a small clinical point? In the last 18 months I have had two patients with an obscure encephalitis and their blood was taken for virus serology, and on both occasions a really significant rise in titre to herpes simplex was reported but in fact both these cases proved to have bacterial endocarditis. I don't know the significance of this. Now may I ask about treatment with idoxuridine? The eye people describe two different pathologies of keratitis. Firstly a direct invasion by the virus and a consequent reaction, and secondly a lesion deep in the cornea which is an immune reaction. I understand that the first type responds to IDU, the second does not. This links up with the comment made by Cutler on the chemotherapy of panencephalitis reported in Neurology (Minneapolis) of January 1968, in a special supplement on measles panencephalitis. He had labelled IDU and had been quite unable to obtain it from the CSF and suggested that it never got through the blood brain barrier. How does this affect our interpretation of results of herpes simplex encephalitis treated with IDU? Is it just the doctor who is being treated? We ourselves perhaps were guilty of this misinterpretation in the two cases we reported from Cardiff. Cutler made a further point that IDU is broken down very rapidly in the brain and again this suggests that it might be of little value in treatment.

MacCallum: Could I try and answer that? If we take the question of the eye infections I am not sure that this is really relevant. In herpes keratitis you have probably got, in the primary infection, injury of a superficial layer of epithelium, and this is where the virus is. IDU has a low solubility, only 0·1 % in the water solution used. This can penetrate the superficial epithelium and affect the virus in those cells, but even here it does not eliminate the virus. There are recurrences; and recurrent lesions involve largely the stroma—the deep cells. This may be partly an allergic reaction but the drug could not penetrate there even if it was going to do much good. However, steroids may be helpful in a stroma lesion, but you may also reactivate virus, so you have got to give the IDU together with steroids. This seems to me to be a slightly different situation and not really comparable to the brain. It has of course been well recognized since the very early work that IDU is broken down: about four hours for complete breakdown. I thought Cutler referred to work in dogs, and I wasn't sure whether he has actually done work of this sort in children. Calabresi and Professor McCollum at Yale also had difficulty in finding IDU in the CSF. However, this may not apply to brain substance with damaged blood vessels and necrosis around the lesions. I do not think I would be deterred by this even though I am not a neurologist. I didn't mention the Cardiff cases in my talk because I felt that treatment had started so late that benefit had really not been achieved. In the Glasgow case there was extreme optimism and enthusiasm, and I felt this had played a part since I find it difficult to believe that the drug could have acted so quickly. I am trying to keep an open mind on this.

DICK: I think Dr MacCallum has made an important point that when the blood barrier is damaged lots of things will get through much more easily. This is shown by Sherwin and other people in Canada in experiments in animals. One warning which I should like to make in the use of antibody and that is the use of falling titres. One sees a number of publications with the diagnosis made on four to eight-fold falling titres. I am very dubious about that and think one has to interpret these results very carefully. Dr Tomlinson's first case was absolutely acceptable. Here there was a falling titre of something from 1000 to 20.

May I ask Dr MacCallum whether he had a chance to do any fractionation of the serum of patients to see whether this might give an index as to whether the infection was a recent primary infection in which one might expect to get more macroglobulin than other globulin in the serum? May I also underline the importance of the number of cases of encephalopathy following pertussis vaccination. I think the numbers are far greater than we know about. Many people including medical officers of health are unwilling to report these from an immunization procedure in which they genuinely believe. There has been a considerable amount of encephalopathy, probably associated with the fact that the pertussis vaccine contained instead of about 20×10^9 micro-organisms, about 29×10^9, and the toxicity is related to the number of micro-organisms. Moreover, the evidence is doubtful that pertussis vaccines do very much good. One last point about steroids: I find it depressing that we have no data yet on the value of steroids. At the Wye meeting four years ago the question was raised, and again last year. But we still have no answer. I think it is important that we do get some accurate data on this. It would provide some index as to whether it might be good to use steroids for all children, say with measles encephalitis. Perhaps enquiring into this would be much better than using vaccine, and the money better spent.

MACCALLUM: May we leave other questions about steroids until after Dr Webb's paper this afternoon?

SPILLANE: A quick question to Dr Bower. One type of acute encephalopathy which I have seen, which you did not mention, is the encephalopathy in a child who has been scalded or burnt. They are quite striking. I have seen one also in an old person whom we thought had a cerebral vascular accident. With no evidence of viral encephalitis presumably these are examples of an acute toxic encephalopathy.

MacCallum: I much regret we are going to have to stop at this stage, but Dr Alpers has a brief announcement.

Alpers: This afternoon I will be talking about Kuru and mentioning the clinical aspects. This is too much to cover in a short time and I have therefore provided some reprints which can be obtained from the office. There is also a protocol put out from Dr Gajdusek's group at the N.I.H. on the collection of specimens for virus isolation. This is an important practical problem because usually by the time these cases have been through the neuropathologist's hands it is too late to get any worthwhile virus specimens.

Slow Virus Diseases of the Nervous System

Chairman
W.McMenemy

Introduction

W. McMenemy

Ladies and gentlemen, I think we must start. We have a full programme this afternoon. It is really in three parts. Firstly we are going to hear about Kuru and Srapie and then about measles and subacute sclerosing panencephalitis and thirdly about the pathogenesis of viral encephalitis and vaccinial reactions. I will call on Dr Alpers to give his paper on Kuru.

Kuru: Clinical and Aetiological Aspects

Michael Alpers

Introduction

Kuru is a subacute degenerative disease of the central nervous system characterized by progressive cerebellar ataxia, a fatal termination, and a natural restriction to the Fore-speaking people of the Eastern Highlands of New Guinea and the neighbours with whom they have inter-married. It apparently began in the region about 60 years ago, and spread from a single focus, slowly at first but with gathering momentum, until it reached epidemic proportions at the time of its discovery by medical science in 1957. The population of all village groups with a history of Kuru is today about 40,000 people and the Kuru region so defined occupies about 1000 square miles at an altitude between 1500 and 2500 metres. Over 80% of cases in all, and virtually all recent cases, have been recorded from the Fore people themselves (population about 14,500). The disease is uniformly fatal and has an average dura-tion of one year: hence the prevalence ratio and the annual incidence and mortality rates work out to be the same: of the order of 1% of the population. The disease predominantly affects adult females; until recently at least, children of both sexes were also affected, but very few adult males (Table 9).

TABLE 9. Total annual mortality from Kuru 1957–1965

Year	Child (< 15)			Adolescent (15–19)			Adult (⩾ 20)			Total
	M	F	T	M	F	T	M	F	T	
1957	22	37	59	10	6	16	1	127	128	203
1958	23	41	64	5	7	12	9	124	133	209
1959	31	40	71	6	7	13	5	131	136	220
1960	24	31	55	8	3	11	7	112	119	185
1961	13	27	40	7	8	15	6	108	114	169
1962	25	11	36	10	9	19	11	85	96	151
1963	12	13	25	5	14	19	3	116	119	163
1964	9	5	14	6	4	10	5	88	93	117
1965	6	3	9	8	4	12	9	82	91	112

M = male, F = female, T = subtotal.

7

A definitive bibliography of Kuru is kept up to date, and revised editions regularly made available (Gajdusek & Alpers 1968). The ethnological (Gajdusek & Zigas 1961, Berndt 1962), social (Glasse Shirley 1964), historical (Mathews 1965, Alpers & Gajdusek 1965, Glasse R. M. 1967) and demographic (Gajdusek, Zigas & Baker 1961, Bennett 1962, McArthur 1964, Alpers & Gajdusek 1965) backgrounds to the disease have been described in a preliminary manner in published papers. Further studies have appeared in mimeographed reports, while an enormous amount of data amassed in the region has not yet been published; such information is extremely valuable from many aspects, but none of it is likely, at this stage, to radically change our thinking about the disease.

Clinical aspects in man

Kuru in the Fore language means trembling with cold or fear, or shaking like long grass in the wind, and is a very apt clinical description of the disease. The Fore have grasped its essence—much more than the first European observers, who were obsessed by one rather grotesque facet of it, and called it 'laughing disease'. The first medical accounts of Kuru in 1957 (Gajdusek & Zigas 1957, Zigas & Gajdusek 1957) were followed by more detailed clinical descriptions (Gajdusek & Zigas 1958, Simpson, Lander & Robson 1959, Gajdusek & Zigas 1959, Zigas & Gajdusek 1959). Rail (1962) gave a summary of his clinical findings, which were in close agreement with the conclusions of Alpers (1964, 1966). More recent clinical accounts have been provided by Hornabrook (1966, 1968). The most significant record of the clinical aspects of Kuru is in the extensive collection of film taken by Gajdusek, Sorenson, Alpers and others (Sorenson & Gajdusek 1966), at present being assembled by Gajdusek & Sorenson into a Research Special Film entitled 'Kuru: a comprehensive assembly of all known cinema of the clinical aspects of Kuru'.

Kuru is essentially a subacute cerebellar degeneration, and the clinical findings, in terms of the primary, progressive and essential signs, are all referable to the cerebellar system. As a description of the full manifestations of the disease, however, this is very inadequate. In terms of its minor signs Kuru is a protean disease of the central nervous system, with involvement of the brain stem, basal ganglia, diencephalon, and cerebrum as well as the cerebellum. Its course is in most cases monotonically progressive, with an average duration of 12 months (range three to 24 months). The course tends to be slower in older people (Alpers 1964a), but there are individual exceptions to this; occasional cases show a remitting and exacerbating course. The clinical picture is essentially the same irrespective of age and sex.

Kuru may be divided into three clinical stages. The first (ambulant) stage includes the prodromal period and ends when the patient is unable to walk without active support; the second (sedentary) stage ends when the patient is unable to remain sitting up without support; the third (tertiary) stage extends into the terminal state and ends with the patient's death.

The prodromal symptoms consist mainly of headache, malaise, and limb pains, occasionally with specific joint pain, and without, as far as can be determined, objective signs. They last on the average for five weeks, and continue into the definitive stage of the disease. They have never been properly explained. At this point, considering the prevalence of Kuru in the region, the patient will suspect the onset of Kuru: because of the non-specific nature of these early symptoms this readily explains many of the reported 'recoveries from Kuru'. Once ataxia begins, however, the patient's self-diagnosis of a fatal disease is likely to be correct. Often the first sign of Kuru, in a person normal to all objective neurological tests, is an unhappy withdrawal from society, and poverty and self-consciousness of movement, brought on by the realization of impending Kuru. Once the ataxia is established the diagnosis is obvious to all, and the patient's reactive depression, in most cases, subsides.

The first symptom proper of Kuru is nearly always unsteadiness in walking. The fundamental signs are postural instability, ataxia of gait and tremor. The incoordination begins in the midline and is shown by marked trunkal instability and astasia; titubation, trunkal tremor and trembling of the legs; and a wide-based, unsteady gait. As the disease progresses the upper limb also becomes involved, and dysmetria, dysdiadochokinesis, decomposition of movement, and intention tremor are found on examination. Every muscle of the body seems eventually to be involved by the ataxic disorganization of movement: facial expression is poorly controlled, extraocular movements are jerky and irregular, and speech is slurred or tremulous. All these signs betoken disease of the cerebellum, at first and most emphatically in the palaeo-cerebellum, later in the neocerebellum. It is the progression in the fundamental signs of postural instability, ataxia of gait and tremor which mark the progression of the disease and on which the division into the three clinical stages is based.

The question of tremor in Kuru is one which has caused some difficulty and embarrassment. The connotation of extra-pyramidal disorder associated with the word 'tremor', despite its much wider denotation, reinforced by the initial description of Kuru as 'resembling paralysis agitans', has made recent workers avoid its use entirely. The phenomenon is quite unmistakable, however, and to avoid the word one has to resort to 'alternating contractions', 'trembling' or 'visible tremulousness' to describe it. Furthermore, the distinctions between the various categories of tremor are confused in the neurological literature. A discussion of this matter in relation to Kuru is attempted by Alpers (1964)*. It is sufficient to say here that tremor in Kuru is postural, that is, essentially ataxic, and an expression of the same underlying motor disability as the ataxia itself. Especially initially, a shivering-like component is also evident, and the tremor is potentiated by cold as well as by supporting a posture. The 'Kuru tremor' disappears in sleep or with complete support of the part in a warm place. In the very late stages of the disease an extra-pyramidal, static tremor occurs in some cases.

Astasia is the first objective sign in Kuru; Romberg's test is usually negative. Patients tend to stand with their legs apart and arms across their chests, in order to keep their balance; in a group they will lean on each other and link arms. Movements leading to instability, such as sitting down, are performed hurriedly. The characteristic gait of Kuru is hesitant, wide-based, and staggering, with irregular placement of the feet and lurching to either side. Some cases show a high steppage, and stamping as the foot is brought down. Associated with the hesitancy there is often a backwards and forwards rocking at the initiation of each step. At first, the gait may appear normal except for the evident concentration involved until a sudden loss of equilibrium sends the patient lurching to the side. Later, in the sedentary stage, though unaided walking is impossible, the exaggerated qualities of the gait disturbance can be seen when the patient is being moved about between two sup-

---

* The classification suggested was:
1 'Resting' tremor
   a quivering (shivering-like)
   b static (parkinsonian) tremor
   c postural tremor (including trunkal tremor and titubation; essentially ataxic)
2 'Action' tremor
   a essential tremor, anxiety tremor
   b flapping (wilsonian) tremor
   c intention tremor (ataxic tremor)

porters. There is marked trunkal instability, weakness at hips and knees and heavy leaning on one or other assistant; such steps as are taken are characterized by jerky, flinging, at times decomposed movements, which lead to a high-steppage, stamping gait. Others may show nothing but a limp drag of their feet; or, in contrast, a stiff shuffling, with rigidity of hips and knees. Occasional cases show scissoring of their legs while being 'walked'.

Once the ambulant stage is passed astasia and gait ataxia can of course no longer be seen, but the progression of the disease may still be noted in the trunk and the arms. For a while the patient is able to sit without support and may continue to take part normally in feasts and meetings, provided someone carries her or assists her to get there. Eventually she passes into the tertiary stage; in this stage she tends to spend her day sitting outside, clutching a stick set up near her house. Finally, even this stick is insufficient support for her and a slight displacement may send her body lurching uncontrollably in the opposite direction in an over-compensated movement. She must then lie down or remain cradled in the arms of a close relative.

Dysarthria is the other early and important progressive sign in the disease. In many cases the speech is high-pitched, thin and tremulous; in others slurred, without changes in pitch or timbre; and in some staccato or scanning. Terminally, speech is lost completely, and dysphagia becomes an added disability.

Other signs which are found in Kuru will now be briefly described. It is important to emphasize that the clinical picture is, in its broad essentials at least, remarkably uniform. However, each case has one or two additional little idiosyncrasies, and if a catalogue of them is given the list becomes disproportionately long; hence a summary will be given only of the more common findings.

The most important are strabismus, clonus and emotional lability. A convergent strabismus is quite common, especially in younger patients. It may begin at any stage of the disease, though it commonly does so early and persists throughout the course; terminally it characteristically disappears. More irregular signs of oculomotor imbalance and incoordination are found in all cases, without the establishment of a permanent strabismus. Ankle and patellar clonus, sometimes with toe and finger clonus as well, is a transient but very striking phenomenon in nearly all cases; it is unassociated with exaggerated tendon reflexes and other signs of pyramidal tract disease. Emotional lability, leading usually to laughing and smiling, but occasionally weeping, is a common but by no means universal finding (about a third of cases show it), occurring in the second or third stage.

Despite the frequency of irregular, jerky eye movements, true nystagmus does not occur in Kuru. Pupillary responses are, with rare exceptions, normal. Photophobia and blepharospasm are common in a mild degree, are occasionally severe and then often asymmetrical. Optic fundi appear normal.

Cranial nerve palsies do not occur in Kuru, though transient supranuclear signs, especially in the later stages, are found. Special senses appear normal.

Asthenia and increased fatiguability of muscles is common and in some cases very marked from an early stage. Paralysis does not occur. Terminally, minimal signs of lower motor neurone disease may be found. Inconsistent pyramidal signs occur, with negative Babinski.

Occasional cases show striking extrapyramidal disorders of posture in the third stage, with dystonic, athetoid or choreiform movements. A static, parkinsonian tremor is also occasionally seen.

With the possible exception of hyperaesthesia in some cases, sensory function remains quite intact.

Passive tone is variable. There is a tendency towards hypotonia early in the course, plastic rigidity around the beginning of the third stage, often with a cogwheel element to it, and terminal flaccidity; but there are many individual exceptions to this. The deep tendon reflexes are equally variable and follow no consistent pattern: they tend to be normal until the third stage, when they become hyperactive, and terminally show a capricious depression; occasionally, primitive reflexes are evident in the terminal state.

Convulsions have never been recorded in Kuru.

Grasp reflexes and associated phenomena may occur in the late stages. Urinary and faecal incontinence is common terminally. Clouding of intellect and consciousness is a terminal finding. Occasional cases show an early and progressive dementia, but what is striking in a terminally incapacitated patient is the relative absence of dementia. Disorders of affect are similarly rare. Most cases view their disease with stoic indifference; some, especially males, become sullen and depressed; a few older women become belligerent. Despite the frequency of emotional lability, the emotional responses characteristically remain appropriate and are not associated with a permanent euphoric mood.

General findings outside the nervous system are unremarkable, except terminally when upper respiratory infection, pneumonia, decubitus ulceration and burns are commonly found.

Terminally, the motor system is generally depressed, except for pseudobulbar signs. The patient is flaccid, mute and emaciated. Infection may hasten the end; but if not, gradual bulbar depression leads to death, which comes very slowly.

Interlude

The pathological findings in Kuru, which show neuronal degeneration, astrocytic hyperplasia, gliosis, and status spongiosus, with minimal demyelination and no inflammatory changes, occur throughout the brain, but especially in the cerebellum. They have been described by Fowler & Robertson (1959), Klatzo, Gajdusek & Zigas (1959), Neumann, Gajdusek & Zigas (1964), Beck & Daniel (1965) and Kakulas, Lecours & Gajdusek (1967).

The first investigations into the aetiology of this new and unusual disease sought to establish a genetic hypothesis (Bennett, Rhodes & Robson 1959) or adopted a many-sided approach (Gajdusek & Zigas 1959, Gajdusek 1963). Early inoculation experiments were unsuccessful, but later, further attempts were made using the chimpanzee as experimental host. In the meantime it seemed that, even though the single gene hypothesis might not necessarily be correct, some genetic predisposition in the Fore people was essential to explain the continued epidemiological findings (Alpers 1965, Mathews 1965). As yet, no convincing evidence has been brought forward to contradict this assertion. In view of the ease with which it could be contradicted, and our failure to do so, despite the continual search for cases of contact transmission in people of established non-Fore ancestry, this requirement must stand for the present.

However, we have now to consider an additional aetiological component: a transmissible, replicating agent. After an incubation period of two years Kuru was successfully transmitted from human brain to the chimpanzee (Gajdusek, Gibbs & Alpers 1966) and, with a reduction of incubation period to one year, passaged from chimpanzee to chimpanzee (Gajdusek, Gibbs & Alpers 1967).

Clinical aspects in the chimpanzee

The chimpanzees were inoculated when about two years old, and thus came down with the disease at the age of three or four. The syndrome has been reproduced with equal ease in both sexes.

The first indication of disease is apathy, lethargy and poverty of movement associated with an increased irritability. This persists for some weeks before more specific signs are noted. Often the first is a fine titubation noted as the animal sits up in the corner of its cage. When the cage door is opened a normal chimpanzee will bound outside: the affected animal remains huddled in a corner with arms across its chest and leans against the cage for support. It characteristically has a vacant expression on its face and a pendulous lower lip. It appears to be abnormally sensitive to cold and widespread pilo-erection is frequently seen. Some animals show a mass reflex akin to the Moro reflex on peripheral stimulation of any sort. Wide grimacing and high-pitched screaming is another reaction to stimulation frequently found.

Unmistakable postural instability and ataxia soon develop. Gait is slow, clumsy and wide-based and attempts to negotiate obstacles in the path lead to wild lurching and falling over. Occasional shivering-like tremors are seen. Hand movements become dysmetric and the animal soon avoids moving its hands at all. One of the most characteristic early signs of the disease is the use of the mouth directly to pick up objects of food, the animal crouching low over the floor in order to do so. There is difficulty in regaining an upright posture when the animal is placed on its back; it soon becomes impossible for it to accomplish this, which provides one convenient test for the degree of progression of the disease. In the early stages of its disability the animal suffers many stumbles and falls. As the disease progresses the degree of postural instability and ataxia increases, until the animal is unable to sit up without support, and has to be hand fed. Decubitus ulceration may develop, and swallowing becomes difficult. In this moribund state the animal is killed for further study. The duration of illness from onset to terminal state varies from three to nine months.

Other signs found include strabismus in a few cases and a marked degree of visual confusion and perseveration of movement. Vision and hearing remain grossly intact. Vestibular function is preserved. Sensory function to pain and touch is preserved; in the later stages there may be hyperaesthesia. Passive tone and deep tendon reflexes remain essentially normal. Plantar reflexes are flexor. Snout reflexes are exaggerated in advanced disease. The optic fundi appear normal. There is no paralysis, and convulsions do not occur. Terminally, the animal is vacuous and confused; but it remains tractable, and learned responses, for example answering to its name, are retained to the end.

Aetiological aspects

The pathology of experimental Kuru in chimpanzees has been reported by Beck, Daniel, Alpers, Gajdusek & Gibbs (1966). It resembles very closely human Kuru, differing only by the greatly increased cortical status spongiosus in the experimental disease. The only other diseases with similar pathology are Scrapie in sheep and encephalopathy in mink. The relationship of Kuru to Scrapie was first appreciated by Hadlow (1959); since then further similarities have been demonstrated, and it is reasonable to assume that the properties of the Kuru agent will be like those of the Scrapie agent. Some concepts of these agents, and slow viruses in general, are briefly discussed at the conclusion of this paper.

Regarding Kuru itself, the general problems relating to its aetiological elucidation have been cogently discussed by Gajdusek (1963). Since then the problems have been clarified somewhat and it now appears that three factors are involved: the transmissible Kuru agent, the genetic background of the Fore people, and, as the means of transmission of the agent, the practice of cannibalism.

The continuing necessity to postulate a genetic predisposition to the disease among the Fore population has already been alluded to. The argument for this depends not on the familial nature of the disease (which might equally have an environmental cause), nor on genetic analysis of pedigrees, but on the absolute limitation of the disease to the Fore people and those related to them genetically, who continue to suffer from Kuru even after migration into new environments, whereas their neighbours, who have essentially the same culture, including the practice of cannibalism, and have undergone similar cultural changes since the irruption of Western civilization into the region in the 1950's, remain free of the disease. This matter is discussed more fully by Alpers & Gajdusek (1965), Alpers (1965, 1967).

The remarkable recent changes in the epidemiological pattern of Kuru may be appreciated from Table 9. These changes are described in more detail in the three papers above, and also in Bennett, Gabb & Oertel (1966) and Gajdusek & Alpers (1966). What has been most striking is the decline in incidence in children, to the extent of total disappearance of the disease in the younger age group. The disease appears to be dying back, as it were, from the youngest age group upwards, in particular amongst those born since 1957 when the area first came under strict government control. Possible environmental changes which may have brought this about are tabulated in Alpers (1965). The change which was most dramatic and which most readily explains the decline in Kuru

is the rapid cessation at this time of the practice of cannibalism. Furthermore, cannibalism would also explain the age and sex incidence as
found in 1957, for the adult males tended not to cannibalize their dead
relatives and, if they did partake, only to eat muscle. The women and
young children of both sexes ate all parts of the body, including brain
and viscera, often inadequately cooked. Cannibalism, therefore, as a
mode of transmission of the agent provides a plausible explanation for
both the initial sex and age distribution and the recent epidemiological
changes. Recent cases are presumably due to the long incubation of the
disease following an exposure before 1957. Background information
on the origin, spread and practice of cannibalism in the Kuru region is
provided by Glasse (1967) and Berndt (1962).

The agent, we must suppose, arose in the region as a mutation, and
may have become further adapted by passage in the human host (Gibbs,
Alpers & Gajdusek 1967). Such mutations are likely to explain the
sporadic outbreaks of familial cerebellar degenerations akin to Kuru
which have been described in other parts of the world (Seitelberger 1962,
Schaltenbrand, Trostdorf, Orthner & Henn 1968). The outbreak in
Kuru we may suppose was much more widespread owing to its occurrence in an established genetic isolate population and to its ability to
spread throughout this population by the practice of cannibalism. It is
conceivable that similar occurrences in the past history of man may
have provided a rational basis for civilized man's apparently inherent
abhorrence of cannibalism.

Regarding the nature of the Kuru agent itself we already have a little
further information. As well as being transmissible and replicating, it
passes a 100 mμ filter, is present in brain to a titre of at least 10^5, can be
transmitted from visceral organs (despite their normal appearance
histologically) and is successfully inoculated via a peripheral route.
Despite many attempts, it has not been seen under the electron microscope; and no evidence for its immunogenicity has yet been produced.
In all these properties it resembles the agent of Scrapie, and experiments
are in progress to characterize it further (Gibbs, Alpers & Gajdusek
1967). Further discussion of its nature depends on analogy with the
Scrapie agent, the remarkable properties of which are described by
others in this Symposium.

In conclusion, some concepts of the possible interaction between
viruses and cells, particularly as they relate to slow virus infections, are
brought forward, in the belief that we must extend the framework of our
thinking if we are to grasp the aetiological possibilities in this field (see

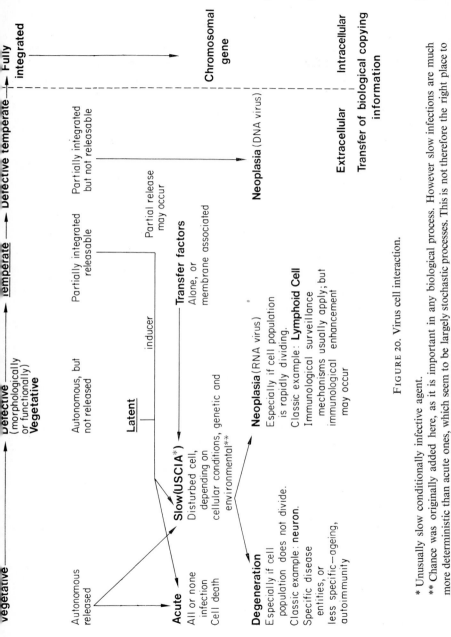

FIGURE 20. Virus cell interaction.

* Unusually slow conditionally infective agent.

** Chance was originally added here, as it is important in any biological process. However slow infections are much more deterministic than acute ones, which seem to be largely stochastic processes. This is not therefore the right place to emphasize chance though it does belong somewhere in the scheme of the figure.

also Gajdusek 1965, 1967). The recent experimental findings in Kuru and Scrapie, and in the related fields of tumour viruses, open up new possibilities in the interaction of viruses and mammalian cells. Many of these findings were foreshadowed by work with the bacteriophages, and it looks now, more and more, that these relationships may have their counterparts in mammalian systems. Figure 20 is offered as a tentative conceptual framework. I shall make no attempt to describe it in detail, or to justify each part of it with the relevant experimental evidence. The framework draws attention to the obvious importance of defectiveness in viral-cell interaction, to the essential similarity of degenerative slow viruses and the RNA tumour viruses, to the possible importance of transfer factors in mediating some of these interactions, and to the closeness of the fully integrated gene to one end of the virus scale. In view of the morphologic connotations of the word 'virus' it might be helpful to think of the interacting agent more as a plasmagene or episome. One studies these agents by their effects, and it is important to realize that there do not really exist rigid entities of 'slow viruses' or 'latent viruses', for example, but rather modes of action with these characteristics. A given agent may be lytic, slow, latent, temperate, or defective, depending on its actual state and mode of action in a given cell. Furthermore, which of these states, be it diseased or normal, which we ascribe to 'viral aetiology' will ultimately depend on our definition of a virus. However, the framework of Fig. 20 is not enhanced by any theoretical discussion. Its function, if it has any at all, is a purely heuristic one.

ACKNOWLEDGEMENTS

Firstly, as always, to Dr Carleton Gajdusek as the source and fountain of our Kuru studies; and to Dr Joseph Gibbs, who has carried the burden of the experimental studies at the National Institute of Neurological Diseases and Blindness in Bethesda. To Dr George Klein of the Department of Tumour Biology, Karolinska Institutet, Stockholm, and to the National Multiple Sclerosis Society of New York, my thanks for their current help and Fellowship support, respectively.

REFERENCES

ALPERS M.P. (1964) *Kuru: a Clinical Study.* Mimeographed. Department of Medicine, University of Adelaide and National Institutes of Health, Bethesda, 38 pp.
ALPERS M.P. (1964a) *Kuru: Age and Duration Studies.* Mimeographed. Department of Medicine, University of Adelaide and National Institutes of Health, Bethesda, 12 pp.

ALPERS M.P. (1965) Epidemiological changes in Kuru, 1957 to 1963. In: *Slow, Latent and Temperate Virus Infections*, NINDB Monograph No. 2, D.C. Gajdusek, C.J. Gibbs, jr & M. Alpers (ed.). Washington D.C. pp. 65–82.

ALPERS M.P. (1966) Kuru. In: *A Manual of Tropical Medicine*, 4th edition, G.W. Hunter, W.W. Frye & J.C. Swartzwelder (eds). Philadelphia, pp. 646–650.

ALPERS M.P. (1967) Kuru: implications of its transmissibility for the interpretation of its changing epidemiological pattern. Presented at the Fifty-sixth Annual Meeting of the International Academy of Pathology, Washington, D.C., March 12–15. To be published in *The Central Nervous System*.

ALPERS M.P. & GAJDUSEK D.C. (1965) Changing patterns of Kuru: epidemiological changes in the period of increasing contact of the Fore people with Western civilization. *Amer. J. trop. Med. Hyg.* **14** : 5, 852–879.

BECK ELISABETH & DANIEL P.M. (1965) Kuru and Scrapie compared: are they examples of system degeneration? In: *Slow, Latent and Temperate Virus Infections*, NINDB Monograph No. 2, D.C. Gajdusek, C.J. Gibbs, jr & M. Alpers (eds). Washington D.C. pp. 85–93.

BECK ELISABETH, DANIEL P.M., ALPERS M., GAJDUSEK D.C. & GIBBS C.J. jr (1966) Experimental 'Kuru' in chimpanzees. A pathological report. *Lancet* ii : 7472, 1056–1059.

BENNETT J.H. (1952) Population studies in the Kuru region of New Guinea. *Oceania*, **33** : 1, 24–46.

BENNETT J.H., GABB B.W. & OERTEL CAROLYN (1966) Further changes of pattern in Kuru. *Med. J. Aust.* i : 10, 379–386.

BENNETT J.H., RHODES F.A. & ROBSON H.N. (1959) A possible genetic basis for Kuru. *Amer. J. hum. Genet.* ii : 2, 169–187.

BERNDT R.M. (1962) *Excess and Restraint. Social Control Among a New Guinea Mountain People.* Chicago, 474 pp.

FOWLER M. & ROBERTSON E.G. (1959) Observations on Kuru. III. Pathological features in five cases. *Australas. Ann. Med.* **8** : 1, 16–26.

GAJDUSEK D.C. (1963) Kuru. *Trans. Roy. Soc. Trop. Med. Hyg.* **57** : 3, 151–169.

GAJDUSEK D.C. (1965) Kuru in New Guinea and the origin of the NINDB study of slow, latent, and temperate virus infections of the nervous system of man. In: *Slow, Latent, and Temperate Virus Infections*, NINDB Monograph No. 2, D.C. Gajdusek, C.J. Gibbs, jr & M. Alpers (eds). Washington, D.C. pp. 3–12.

GAJDUSEK D.C. (1967) Slow virus infections of the nervous system. *New Eng. J. Med.* **276** : 7, 392–400.

GAJDUSEK D.C. & ALPERS M.P. (1966) Kuru in childhood: disappearance of the disease in the younger age group. *J. Pediat.* **69** : 5, Pt 2, 886–887.

GAJDUSEK D.C. & ALPERS M.P. (1968) *Bibliography of Kuru.* Mimeographed. National Institutes of Health, Bethesda, 79 pp.

GAJDUSEK D.C., GIBBS C.J. jr & ALPERS M. (1966) Experimental transmission of a Kuru-like syndrome to chimpanzees. *Nature*, **209** : 5025, 794–796.

GAJDUSEK D.C., GIBBS C.J. jr & ALPERS M. (1967) Transmission and passage of experimental 'Kuru' to chimpanzees. *Science*, **155** : 3759, 212–214.

GAJDUSEK D.C. & ZIGAS V. (1957) Degenerative disease of the central nervous system in New Guinea. The endemic occurrence of 'Kuru' in the native population. *New Eng. J. Med.* 257: 30, 974–978.

GAJDUSEK D.C. & ZIGAS V. (1958) Untersuchungen über die Pathogenese von Kuru: eine klinische, pathologische und epidemiologische Untersuchung einer chronischen, progressiven, degenerativen und unter den Eingeborenen der Eastern Highlands von Neu Guinea epidemische Ausmasse erreichenden Erkrankung des Zentralnervensystems. *Klin. Wschr.* **36** : 10, 445–459.

GAJDUSEK D.C. & ZIGAS V. (1959) Kuru. Clinical, pathological and epidemiological study of an acute progressive degenerative disease of the central nervous system among natives of the Eastern Highlands of New Guinea. *Amer. J. Med.* **26** : 3, 442–469.

GAJDUSEK D.C. & ZIGAS V. (1961) Studies on Kuru. I. The ethnologic setting of Kuru. *Amer. J. trop. Med. Hyg.* **10** : 1, 80–91.

GAJDUSEK D.C., ZIGAS V. & BAKER J. (1961) Studies on Kuru. III. Patterns of Kuru incidence: demographic and geographic epidemiological analysis. *Amer. J. trop. Med. Hyg.* **10** : 4, 599–627.

GIBBS C.J. jr, ALPERS M. & GAJDUSEK D.C. (1967) Attempts to transmit subacute and chronic neurological diseases to animals. With a progress report on the experimental transmission of Kuru to chimpanzees. Presented at the Workshop on Contributions to the Pathogenesis and Etiology of Demyelinating Diseases, Locarno, Switzerland, May 31–June 3. To be published in Proceedings.

GLASSE R.M. (1967) Cannibalism in the Kuru region of New Guinea. *Trans. N.Y. Acad. Sci.* **29** : 6, 748–754.

GLASSE SHIRLEY (1964) The social effects of Kuru. *Papua N.G. Med. J.* **7** : 1, 36–47.

HADLOW W.J. (1959) Scrapie and Kuru. *Lancet* ii : 7097, 289–290.

HORNABROOK R.W. (1966) A review of the clinical features of Kuru. In: *Proceedings of the Fifth International Congress of Neuropathology, Zurich, Aug. 31–Sept. 3, 1965*, F.Lüthy & A.Bischoff (eds). Excerpta Medica Foundation, Amsterdam, pp. 211–212.

HORNABROOK R.W. (1968) Kuru—a subacute cerebellar degeneration. The natural history and clinical features. *Brain*, **91** : 1, 53–74.

KAKULAS B.A., LECOURS A.-R. & GAJDUSEK D.C. (1967) Further observations on the pathology of Kuru (a study of the two cerebra in serial section). *J. Neuropath. exp. Neurol.* **26** : 1, 85–97.

KLATZO I., GAJDUSEK D.C. & ZIGAS V. (1959) Pathology of Kuru. *Lab. Invest.* **8** : 4, 799–847.

MATHEWS J.D. (1965) The changing face of Kuru. An analysis of pedigrees collected by R.M.Glasse and Shirley Glasse and of recent census data. *Lancet*, i : 7396, 1138–1141.

MCARTHUR Norma (1964) The age incidence of Kuru. *Ann. hum. Genet.* **27**, 341–352.

NEUMANN META, GAJDUSEK D.C. & ZIGAS V. (1964) Neuropathologic findings in exotic neurologic disorders among natives of the highlands of New Guinea. *J. Neuropath. exp. Neurol.* **23** : 3, 486–507.

RAIL L. (1962) Further investigations into Kuru. Presented at the First Asian and Oceanian Congress of Neurology, Tokyo, October 7–10. Mimeographed. National Institutes of Health, Bethesda.

SCHALTENBRAND G., TROSTDORF E., ORTHNER H. & HENN R. (1968) Kuruähnliche sklerosierende panencephalomyelitis in Europa. *Deutsch. Z. Nervenheilk.* **193** : 2, 158–194.

SEITELBERGER F. (1962) Eigenartige familiärhereditäre Krankheit des Zentralnerven-systems in einer niederösterreichischen Sippe (Zugleich ein Beitrag zur vergleich-enden Neuropathologie des Kuru). *Wien. Klin. Wschr.* **74** : 41–42, 687–691.

SIMPSON D. A., LANDER H. & ROBSON H. N. (1959) Observations on Kuru. II. Clinical features. *Australas. Ann. Med.* **8** : 1, 8–15.

SORENSEN E. R. & GAJDUSEK D. C. (1966) The study of child behavior and develop-ment in primitive cultures. A research archive for ethnopediatric film investiga-tions of styles in the patterning of the nervous system. *Pediatrics,* **37** : 1, Pt 2, 149–243.

ZIGAS V. & GAJDUSEK D. C. (1957) Kuru: clinical study of a new syndrome resembling paralysis agitans in natives of the Eastern Highlands of Australian New Guinea. *Med. J. Aust.* ii : 21, 745–754.

ZIGAS V. & GAJDUSEK D. C. (1959) Kuru: clinical, pathological and epidemiological study of a recently discovered acute progressive degenerative disease of the central nervous system reaching 'epidemic' proportions among natives of the Eastern Highlands of New Guinea. *Papua N.G. Med. J.* **3** : 1, 1–24.

Scrapie—Natural and Experimental

H. B. Parry

Scrapie is a spontaneous subacute progressive neuromyopathic degeneration of sheep, associated with a transmissible agent (TSA) capable on inoculation into experimental animals of causing a somewhat similar syndrome, which, although frequently called Scrapie, is more accurately termed experimental Scrapie encephalopathy.

Natural Scrapie has been known for two centuries, its aetiology in dispute (see Parry 1957, 1962, Palmer 1959). Recent studies of the experimental disease have led to the proposal that Scrapie is a slow virus infection, a view which is difficult to reconcile with much relevant evidence on natural Scrapie. Indeed Scrapie is probably an example of a more novel biological situation: a gene controlled abiotrophy or degeneration of the central nervous system in middle age which is mediated through or closely associated with an internally generated and self-replicating agent transmissible and encephalopathogenic experimentally. The agent is not an infectious virus (Parry 1962, 1964b), but a provirus of an unusual type, whose novel features Hunter (1968) and Haig (1968) and their colleagues are now defining.

The biological parameters of natural Scrapie have many features in common with a number of degenerative neurological disorders in man (Parry 1962, Gibbs & Gajdusek 1965). These include Kuru (Alpers 1968), and a number of multiple system atrophies of middle age such as the subacute presenile encephalopathies (Nevin 1967). Creutzfeldt-Jakob disease (Brownell & Oppenheimer 1965) and Schut's hereditary progressive ataxias (Schut 1951) and other olivo-ponto-cerebellar atrophies may also fall into this general category.

1 Natural Scrapie of sheep

This is an hereditary probably non-infectious fatal disease of sheep in middle age affecting both sexes equally, due to a bilaterally symmetrical primary degeneration of the olivo-ponto-cerebellar, and hypothalamo-neurohypophyseal systems (Beck, Daniel & Parry 1964). The main clinical signs are related to (1) locomotor incoordination, ataxia, tremor and asthenia, (2) hypothalamic dysfunction affecting metabolism and body

8

homeostasis, temperature control and cardiovascular stability, (3) constant rubbing suggestive of sensory disturbance, (4) behavioural disorders with emotional instability and (5) defects of vision (Parry 1957, 1962). Its pattern of occurrence is compatible with a hereditary disease, controlled by a simple autosomal recessive gene with full penetrance (Parry 1960, 1962, Draper & Parry 1962), which can give rise to outbreaks of disease resembling infectious epidemics (Draper 1963) such as have been frequently noted in the field. The TSA is present in the hereditary cases (Parry 1962), shortly before and during the clinical illness. Repeated attempts to demonstrate communicability of the disease by introducing sheep from unaffected flocks to affected flocks and *vice versa* have revealed no evidence to support the view that natural Scrapie is ever transmitted in the field by an infectious agent through contact, coitus, gestation, suckling, contaminated surroundings or intermediate vectors (Parry 1962, 1964a, b).

2   The hereditary basis of Scrapie

Reasonable proof that a disease affecting a large mammal in middle age is due to a recessive gene requires quantitative data suitable for rigorous statistical analysis (Draper & Parry 1962, Draper 1963). Five main criteria must be met: (1) Establish that the epidemiological and general clinico-pathological data are compatible and recognize individuals of the three possible genotypes—*SS* & *Ss* (unaffected) and *ss* (affected). (2) Determine the ratios of affected to unaffected in matings of known genotypes. (3) Demonstrate that progeny with one homozygous dominant *SS* parent are *always* unaffected. (4) Develop a population virtually free of gene *s*, in which the disease does not occur. (5) Where an infectious agent may be involved, the data for criteria 2, 3 and 4 are crucial and must be assembled under conditions fully congenial to manifestation of the disease, i.e. in a community affected continuously during the period of observation.

These criteria have been met for Scrapie, except for the final phase of criterion 4.

The data have been assembled in a nearly-closed breeding population of 20,000 sheep under close supervision for 15 years (six to eight generations) in which 2000 cases of Scrapie have been observed. In two flocks of 1500 sheep providing crucial information meeting criterion 5, most animals whether affected or not have been autopsied and their brains examined histopathologically, before a final diagnosis is declared.

The evidence for criteria 1 and 2 have been published (Parry 1957,

1960, 1962, Draper & Parry 1962). For criterion 3, 23 rams have been test-mated to establish that they are of *SS* genotype. Eight have been found (*P* < 1 : 100). None of the 250 progeny of these rams has been affected whatever the Scrapie status of their other parent (see Table 10), or of the 10 flocks in which they have been born, reared and lived until four and a half years old or more.

TABLE 10. Sheep born, reared and kept in a high incidence Scrapie flock

Sire: proven *SS* ram Dam's status:	No. of Progeny surviving to age (years)				
	0·75	4·5	5·5	8·5	10·5
ss—affected during its gestation and suckling	13	11	9	2	1
ss—affected later	14	10	10	4	1
Ss—unaffected	29	23	20	4	1
Ss/SS unaffected	34	24	14		
TOTAL	90	68	53	10	3
Scrapie affected	0	0	0	0	0

Criterion 4 has been met in part. Seven proven-*SS* rams have been used over a decade in one flock, in which 40–55 % of the cohort (females born in one year retained in the flock) for several years were dying of Scrapie. The introduction of the progeny of these *SS* rams, while deliberately breeding some *ss* and *sS* individuals in each cohort, has been accompanied by a reduction of Scrapie to < 1 %, at which level it is being maintained (see Figure 21). The final stage of developing a gene-free (*P* < 1 : 1000) sheep population in which random mating can be allowed without Scrapie recurring, depends on the use over four to five successive generations of proven *SS* sires, to produce sheep designated as 4 or 5W. A small number of 4W individuals are now available with several hundred 2W and 3W sheep. A further five years should allow completion of the final prediction. The present evidence offers substantial proof that the manifestation of natural Scrapie is determined solely by an autosomal recessive gene or a mechanism indistinguishable at present therefrom.

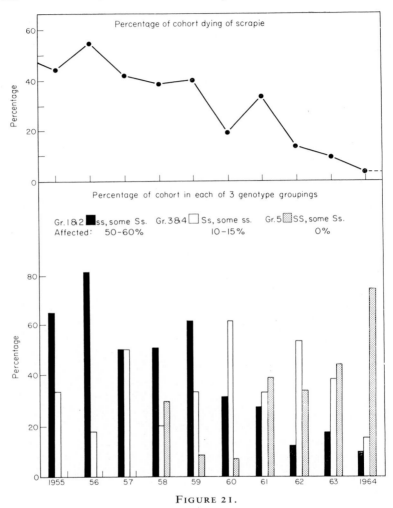

FIGURE 21.

Deaths from scrapie in one flock over a decade and their relation to the genotype composition of the cohorts born in successive years.

3 *Experimental Scrapie encephalopathy (ESE) and the transmissible agent (TSA)*

The principal features of experimental Scrapie following injections of tissue extracts etc. are well known (see Gajdusek *et al.* 1965), and it is commonly equated with natural Scrapie. However the experimental disease has certain properties, which distinguish it from the natural and justify the separate designation experimental Scrapie encephalopathy (ESE): (1) the clinical syndrome of ESE in sheep is often quite distinct from the natural one; (2) the diffuse glial proliferation and extensive status spongiosus are much more extensive in ESE, particularly in the forebrain which is spared in the natural disease. (3) ESE may be transmitted by ingestion, occasionally by contact and across the placenta, not so natural Scrapie. (4) ESE is probably not transmitted through the genetic mechanism, and susceptibility to TSA is not co-terminous with any natural scrapie genotype. (5) ESE can be induced by the injection of TSA-active material from sources other than natural Scrapie, e.g. human multiple sclerosis (Campbell *et al.* 1963, Pálsson *et al.* 1965, Field 1966), epidemic encephalopathy of mink (Burger & Hartsough 1965, Zlotnik & Barlow 1967), normal mice and mice bearing tumours (Pattison & Jones 1968).

Thus experimental Scrapie encephalopathy is a separate disease entity caused by transmissible agents from a variety of natural sources. It should be considered as an example of a group of *subacute experimental encephalopathies* caused by a special type of *transmissible encephalopathic agent* (TEPA), which occur in a variety of natural situations, usually, as far as it is at present known, associated with, but not confined to, degenerative non-inflammatory disorders of the nervous system. The present arch-type of a TEPA is the Scrapie agent, which is a non-infectious 'non-virus'. The view that Scrapie is a slow virus infection (Gajdusek 1965), i.e. a conventional communicable disease with a long incubation period, is no longer compatible with all the facts; it may be profitable to review the interpretations of human disorders, which have been based on this assumption.

4   *The Scrapie gene and the transmissible agent*
There is no satisfactory evidence that the Scrapie gene acts through an all-or-none susceptibility to an environmental agent, which would have to be ubiquitous. There is a great deal of data against any widespread infection, and no unequivocal evidence in support of the contention.

TSA has only been demonstrated in sheep with clinical Scrapie or shortly before when brain lesions may be demonstrated by light microscopy. TSA has not been demonstrated in normal unaffected sheep.

While no detailed study of TSA in sheep of known genotype has yet been attempted, our present knowledge is that TSA is produced in the *ss* genotype only when degeneration of the CNS has already commenced;

there is no unequivocal evidence that the presence of the agent ever precedes the degeneration.

TSA is not produced in sheep of *SS* and *Ss* genotypes, although some animals of these genotypes are almost certainly able to sustain the replication of inoculated TSA.

Thus a 'substrate-system' suitable for the initial production and replication (probably) of TSA occurs in the *ss*-genotype, while in *SS* and *Ss* genotypes the 'substrate-system' supports replication only.

This 'substrate-system' is probably widespread in many body tissues, most of which are able to harbour TSA without apparent ill-effects. It is only upon certain specialized cells of the CNS that the potential lethal cytopathogenic effects of TSA are manifested.

In natural Scrapie, sheep acquire TSA entirely through heredity and never by infection, although the lethal effect of the gene is long delayed.

The doom of the Scrapie adult is engraved irrevocably on the zygote; the transmissible agent is but a product of this determination.

This work has been supported by grants from the National Foundation for Neuromuscular Diseases of New York.

REFERENCES

ALPERS M. (1968) Kuru. *This Symposium*, pp. 83–97.

BECK E., DANIEL P.M. & PARRY H.B. (1964) Degeneration of the cerebellar and hypothalamo-neurohypophysial systems in sheep with Scrapie; and its relationship to human system degenerations. *Brain* **87**, 153–176.

BROWNELL B. & OPPENHEIMER D. (1965) An ataxic form of subacute presenile polioencephalopathy (Creutzfeldt-Jakob disease). *J. Neurol. Neurosurg. Psych.* **28**, 350–361.

BURGER D. & HARTSOUGH G.R. (1965) Encephalopathy of Mink. II. Experimental and natural transmission. *J. inf. Dis.* **115**, 393–399.

CAMPBELL A.M.G., NORMAN R.M. & SANDRY R.J. (1963) Subacute encephalitis in an adult associated with necrotizing myelitis and results of animal inoculation experiments. *J. Neurol. Neurosurg. Psychiat.* **26**, 439–446.

DRAPER G.J. (1963) 'Epidemics' caused by a late-manifesting gene. Application to Scrapie. *Heredity*, **18**, 165–171.

DRAPER G.J. & PARRY H.B. (1962) Scrapie in sheep; the hereditary component in a high incidence environment. *Nature (Lond.)*, **195**, 670–672.

FIELD E.J. (1966) Transmission experiments with multiple sclerosis: An interim report. *Brit. med. J.* ii, 564–565.

GAJDUSEK D.C., GIBBS C.J., JR, ALPERS M. (eds.) (1965) *Slow, Latent and Temperate Virus Infections.* U.S. Pub. Health Serv. Wash. Pub. No. 1378, N.I.N.D.B. Monograph No. 2., pp. xx and 489.

GAJDUSEK D.C. (1965) *Kuru in New Guinea and the Origin of the NINDB Study of Slow, Latent and Temperate Virus Infections of the Nervous System of Man.* U.S. Pub. Health Serv. Wash. Pub. No. 1378, NINDB Monograph No. 2., pp. 3–13.

GIBBS C.J. JR & GAJDUSEK D.C. (1965) *Attempt to Demonstrate a Transmissible Agent in Kuru, Amyotrophic Laterol Sclerosis, and other Subacute and Chronic Progressive Nervous System Degenerations of Man.* U.S. Pub. Health Serv. Wash. Pub. No. 1378, NINDB Monograph No. 2., pp. 39–48.

HAIG D.A. (1968) The virology of Scrapie. *This Symposium,* pp. 129–131.

HUNTER G.D. (1968) The chemical nature of the scrapie agent. *This Symposium,* pp. 123–128.

NEVIN S. (1967) On some aspects of cerebral degeneration in later life. *Proc. roy. Soc. Med.* **60,** 517–526.

PALMER A.C. (1959) Scrapie: a review of the literature. *Vet. Rev. Anot.* **5,** 1–15.

PÁLSSON P.A., PATTISON I.H. & FIELD E.J. (1965) Tranmission experiments with multiple sclerosis. *Slow, Latent and Temperate Virus Infections,* Gajdusek *et al.* (eds.) pp. 49–54.

PARRY H.B. (1957) Scrapie and related myopathies in sheep. Preliminary observations on their investigation and attempted control by a voluntary health scheme. *Vet. Rec.* **69,** 43–55.

PARRY H.B. (1960) Scrapie: a transmissible hereditary disease of sheep. *Nature (Lond.),* **185,** 441–443.

PARRY H.B. (1962) Scrapie: A transmissible and hereditary disease of sheep. *Heredity,* **17,** 75–105.

PARRY H.B. (1964a) Natural Scrapie of sheep: its occurrence and dissemination in the field. II. The general pattern of occurrence in parts of Great Britain. *Rep. Scrapie Seminar, Washington, D.C.,* 1964. *U.S. Dep. Agric., ARS* 91–53, pp. 120–124.

PARRY H.B. (1964b) The hereditary mechanism in the causation of natural Scrapie in sheep. IV. The possible relationships of the transmissible Scrapie agent (provirus) to the genetical component. *U.S. Dep. Agric., ARS* 91–53, pp. 168–170.

PATTISON I.H. & JONES K.M. (1968) Detection of the Scrapie agent in tissues of normal mice and in tumours of tumour-bearing but otherwise normal mice. *Nature (Lond.),* **218,** 102–104.

SCHUT J.W. (1951) Hereditary ataxia. A survey of certain clinical, pathologic and genetic features with linkage data on five additional hereditary factors. *Amer. J. hum. Genet.* **3,** 93–110.

ZLOTNIK I. & BARLOW R.M. (1967) Transmission of the specific encephalopathy of mink to the goat. *Vet. Rec.* **81,** 55–56.

Similarities and Differences in the Pattern of the Pathological Changes in Scrapie, Kuru, Experimental Kuru and Subacute Presenile Polioencephalopathy

Elisabeth Beck, P. M. Daniel, D. C. Gajdusek
and C. J. Gibbs Jr

The pathological changes in natural Scrapie (Bertrand, Carré & Lucam 1937, Beck, Daniel & Parry 1964), Kuru (Klatzo, Gajdusek & Zigas 1959, Fowler & Robertson 1959, Beck & Daniel 1965a), experimental Kuru (Beck, Daniel, Alpers, Gajdusek & Gibbs 1966), and the ataxic form of subacute presenile polioencephalopathy (Brownell & Oppenheimer 1965) have been fully described in the literature. The purpose of the present paper is to compare and contrast the principal neuropathological changes which occur in these diseases.

Scrapie
We have investigated the brains of 34 sheep suffering from Scrapie; of these 18 were moribund, eight in advanced and another eight in early stages of the disease. The average duration of the illness was six months.

Macroscopically the brains looked normal, microscopically there was a degeneration of the cerebellum and its connexions, of the hypothalamo-neurohypophysial system and in addition there were more generalized changes in the rest of the brain. The severity of the degeneration varied from case to case. In the cerebellum there was patchy loss of Purkinje cells and of granule cells (Fig. 22A) with empty baskets, torpedos and fibrous gliosis (Fig. 23A). No demyelination was seen (Fig. 24A), although there was some neutral fat and subcortical fibrous gliosis. In four cases there were PAS positive plaques. In the brainstem there was generalized proliferation of astrocytes (Fig. 25A), neuronal loss in the nuclei pontis and in other nuclei with cerebellar connexions; there was also vacuolation of many surviving neurones. These nuclei showed marked fibrous gliosis which was confined to their territory. In the hypothalamus there was loss of nerve cells in the supraoptic and paraventricular nuclei with abnormalities in the amount of neurosecretory material within the median eminence. Throughout, the cortical archi-

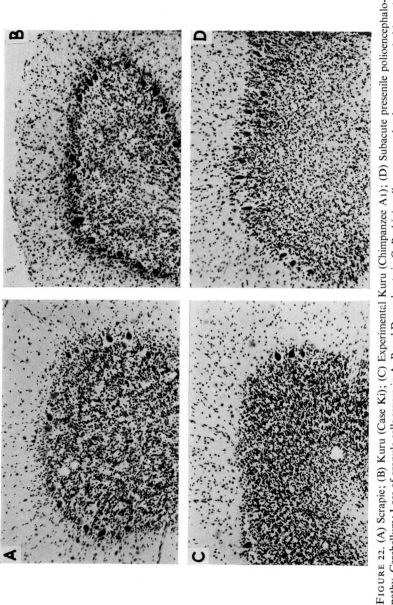

FIGURE 22. (A) Scrapie; (B) Kuru (Case Ki); (C) Experimental Kuru (Chimpanzee A1); (D) Subacute presenile polioencephalopathy. Cerebellum: Loss of granule cells severe in A, B and D, moderate in C; Purkinje cells are somewhat better preserved although many are degenerating with axonal torpedos and swollen dendrites (not illustrated). The number of cells in the molecular layer is greatly increased, particularly in B, C and D and the Bergmann glial cells are proliferated. Nissl stain ×80.

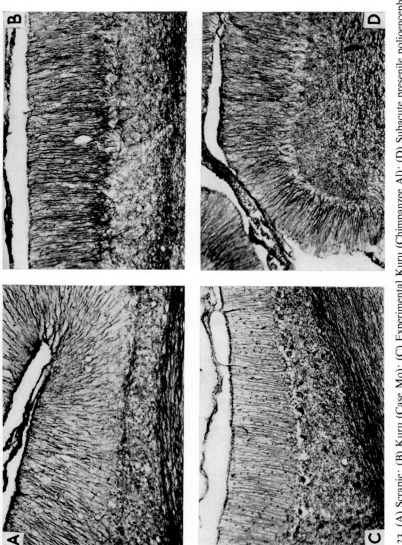

FIGURE 23: (A) Scrapie; (B) Kuru (Case Mo); (C) Experimental Kuru (Chimpanzee Al); (D) Subacute presenile polioencephalo-pathy. Cerebellum: Fibrous gliosis throughout all layers of the cerebellar cortex, severe in A, B and D, moderate in C. The subcortical white matter (shown in A, B and C) was also gliosed. Holzer stain ×80.

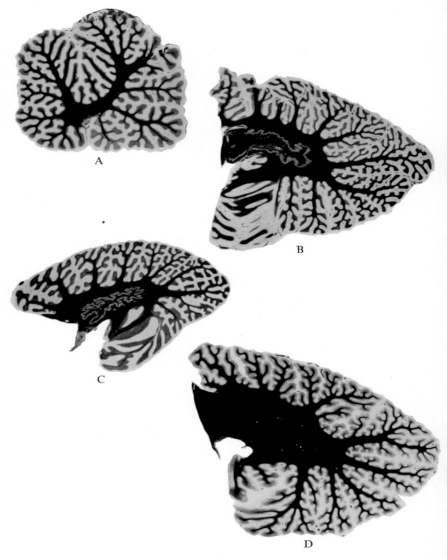

FIGURE 24. (A) Scrapie; (B) Kuru (Case Ki); (C) Experimental Kuru (Chimpanzee Al); (D) Subacute presenile polioencephalopathy. Cerebellum: The cerebellar white matter does not appear demyelinated, although some myelin break-down, secondary to degeneration of neurons in the cerebellar cortex, had occurred. Woelke's modification of Heidenhain's method   ×1·5.

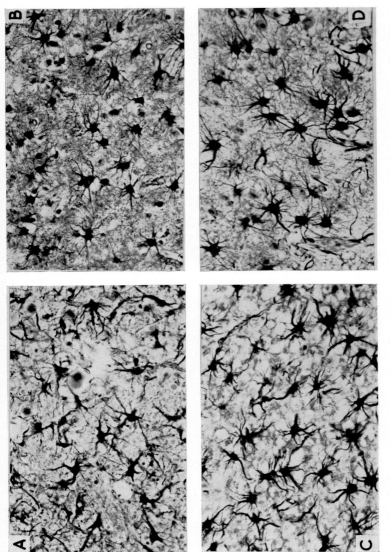

FIGURE 25. (A) Scrapie; (B) Kuru (Case Ki); (C) Experimental Kuru (Chimpanzee A15); (D) Subacute presenile polioencephalopathy. Proliferated and hypertrophic astrocytes in midbrain (A), central cortex (B), occipital cortex (C) and insula cortex (D). Cajal's gold sublimate impregnation ×200.

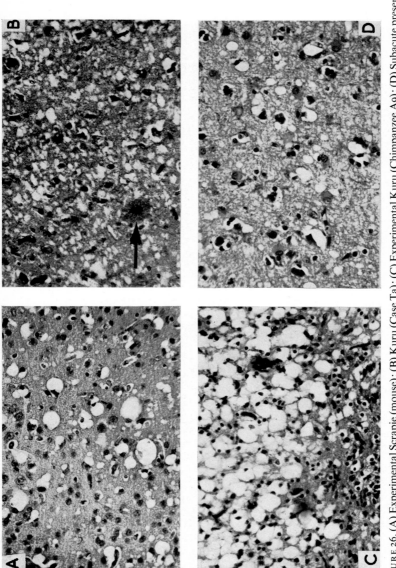

FIGURE 26. (A) Experimental Scrapie (mouse); (B) Kuru (Case Ta); (C) Experimental Kuru (Chimpanzee A9); (D) Subacute presenile polioencephalopathy. Status spongiosus in the cerebral cortex. This does not occur in natural Scrapie, but is well developed in the experimental condition (A); in Kuru it is often confined to cortex belonging to the limbic system (gyrus cinguli B); 'Kuru plaques' (arrow) are frequently found in spongy areas. In experimental Kuru it is most severe and affects the whole of the cerebral gray matter; it is generally less developed in areas containing many myelinated nerve fibres as in the stripe of Genari of the visual cortex (Bottom of Figure C); in polioencephalopathy its development varies between cases. In the present case it was easily recognized in less severely

tecture was preserved, although in places there was a slight proliferation of astrocytes in the deep layers.

Amongst the many authors who have studied experimental Scrapie the papers by Hadlow (1961) on the disease in goats and those by Pattison & Smith (1963) and Pattison (1965) in goats, mice and a number of other laboratory animals should be consulted. We ourselves have not had extensive experience with this disease (Beck & Daniel 1965b), but have been impressed by the degeneration in the cerebellum and in the hypothalamus as well as by status spongiosus of the gray matter (Fig. 26A) and by the widespread proliferation and hypertrophy of astrocytes. These latter changes contrast with the findings in the natural disease and it is of interest that, although status spongiosus does not occur in natural Scrapie, it is a prominent feature in the experimentally induced condition.

Kuru

The first comprehensive neuropathological report of Kuru was published in 1959 by Klatzo, Gajdusek and Zigas, and was based on 12 of the 150 patients reported in the first clinical study by Zigas & Gajdusek (1957). Smaller groups of five and three cases, respectively, were recorded by Fowler & Robertson (1959) and by Neumann, Gajdusek & Zigas (1964). All these investigators are agreed that Kuru belongs to the group of subacute degenerative conditions of the central nervous system. It has been compared with Creutzfeldt-Jakob disease by Klatzo *et al.* (1959) and by Neumann *et al.* (1964), with the subacute cerebellar degenerations by ourselves (1965a) and with olivo-ponto-cerebellar degeneration by Shiraki (1966).

We have examined 13 cases of Kuru; four male and nine female. The age of onset was between four and a half and 30 years with an average of $14\frac{1}{2}$ years. The duration of the illness ranged from five to $13\frac{1}{2}$ months with an average of nine months. Macroscopically the cerebral hemispheres showed no abnormality while the cerebellum regularly showed atrophy which was often severe especially in the paleocerebellum. Microscopically the pathological changes were much the same throughout our 13 cases. In the cerebellum there was loss and degeneration of both Purkinje and granule cells (Fig. 22B) with massive proliferation of microglial cells which were found in all stages of phagocytic activity. Many of the surviving Purkinje cells had torpedos on their axons and had thickened dendrites. Astrocytes had proliferated and there was a dense fibrous gliosis throughout (Fig. 23B). PAS positive plaques were found in three quarters of our cases. Fibrous gliosis and some myelin break-down had also occurred in the cerebellar white matter, although the myelin was not obviously thinned on macroscopic examination of stained sections (Fig. 24B). In the brainstem there was neuronal loss and degeneration and there was also fibrous gliosis in the pontine nuclei, the inferior olives and other nuclei with cerebellar connexions. In about half of our cases the cortico-spinal tracts were degenerated and there was also some degeneration of the spinocerebellar tracts. The median eminence contained an excess of neurosecretory material suggesting an abnormality in the hypothalamo-neurohypophysial system. Another finding in most of our cases was a coarse, often multi-locular vacuolation of the large nerve cells in caudate nucleus and puta-men. In addition there were widespread generalized changes in the cerebral hemispheres. The most striking of these was a mild status spongiosus in limited parts of the cortex and basal ganglia in seven out of the 13 cases (Fig. 26B). In the spongy areas there was always an excess of hypertrophic astrocytes (Fig. 25B) and often rod-shaped microglial cells. There was nerve cell loss which, together with the glial proliferation, tended to obliterate the cytoarchitectonic pattern. Very occasionally there was slight perivascular cuffing of a blood vessel. In the underlying white matter a few vessels would show an accumulation of neutral fat, but, as in the cerebellum, there was no obvious demyel-ination. When status spongiosus was present it was frequently found in the limbic and paralimbic cortices as first pointed out by Kakulas, Lecours & Gajdusek (1967). In all cases, however, there were large areas of cortex where status spongiosus was not obvious and where the cytoarchitecture was well preserved. Of the basal ganglia, apart from the changes mentioned before, the pallidum was relatively well preserved, but the thalamus often showed degeneration with neuronal loss, status spongiosus and severe astrocytic proliferation. Of all the thalamic nuclei, the anterior nuclear complex which belongs to the limbic system was generally the most severely affected. Similarities between Kuru and Scrapie have previously been pointed out (Hadlow 1959, Beck & Daniel 1965a, Beck, Daniel & Gajdusek 1966).

Experimental Kuru

We have examined the brains and spinal cords of 15 chimpanzees. These included the original eight animals which were inoculated intracere-brally with brain suspension from seven different Kuru patients; they also included six animals of the first and one of the second chimpanzee to chimpanzee passage. Amongst the latter there was one chimpanzee which received the inoculum only by a peripheral (not intracerebral) route. The pathological changes found in the brains were essentially the same in every case and this applies not only to the first eight chimpanzees but also to the animals of the first and second passage, whether the inoculum was diluted or filtered, or was given intracerebrally or by the peripheral route. Macroscopically the brains appeared normal but they showed the most remarkable microscopic changes. There was a severe status spongiosus which had destroyed most of the grey matter of the brain (Fig. 26C). In the cerebral hemisphere the spongy state was most marked in the granular cortex and in the striatum, the agranular areas of the cortex and the rest of the basal ganglia being somewhat better preserved. Together with status spongiosus went a massive degeneration and loss of neurones with severe disorganization of the cytoarchitecture and marked proliferation and hypertrophy of astrocytes (Fig. 25C). The white matter was not obviously thinned (Fig. 27), nevertheless microscopically extensive breakdown of myelin was seen and neutral fat was present throughout. An occasional cuffed vessel was seen in two of the 15 cases. The hypothalamo-neurohypophysial system showed slight abnormalities (see Table 11). In the brainstem and cerebellum status spongiosus was minimal; other degenerative changes in these regions closely resembled those seen in natural Kuru, although they were on the whole of lesser severity (Fig. 22C, 23C, 24C).

Subacute presenile polioencephalopathy
While the basic similarities between experimental and human Kuru are obvious, the remarkable status spongiosus in the chimpanzee's brain suggests a further link with still another subacute degeneration of the human brain, that is with the ataxic form of subacute presenile polio-encephalopathy. This term was introduced by Brownell & Oppenheimer (1965) as a nosological entity within the Creutzfeldt-Jakob syndrome and distinct from subacute spongiform encephalopathy, Nevin-Jones disease (1954, 1960). Despite Brownell & Oppenheimer's classification some confusion seems to persist about the differential diagnosis of these two conditions. This is not the place to try to unravel controversial views, our only intention is to present the neuropathological changes found in one case of subacute presenile polioencephalopathy, since a cortical biopsy taken from the patient's brain induced a similar fatal encephalopathy in a chimpanzee, 13 months after intracerebral inoculation.

9

The clinical details of the case will be given by Dr Matthews. The patient's cerebrum and cerebellum showed severe macroscopic atrophy. Microscopically in the cerebellum there was a considerable loss of granule cells with somewhat better preservation of Purkinje cells

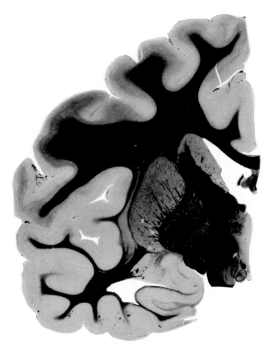

FIGURE 27. Experimental Kuru (Chimpanzee A4). Cerebral hemisphere. The cerebral white matter does not appear demyelinated although considerable myelin breakdown with the formation of neutral fat (not illustrated) was seen. This appears to be secondary to degeneration of neurones within the entire cerebral mantle. Woelke's modification of Heidenhain's method × 1·5.

(Fig. 22D), there were fat-laden microglial cells in the molecular layer and an intense fibrous gliosis was seen throughout (Fig. 23D). The cerebellar white matter appeared normal (Fig. 24D). In contrast to Kuru the changes were equally severe in both paleo- and neocerebellum. In the brainstem the pontine nuclei and inferior olives were preserved, but

TABLE 11. Similarities and differences in the pattern of the pathological changes in Scrapie, Kuru, experimental Kuru and subacute presenile polioencephalopathy

	Peri-vascular cuffing	Coarsely vacuol. neurones	Hypertr. Prolifer. astrocytes	Status spongiosus	Cortical architecture	White matter	Cerebellum paleocer.	neocer.	PAS positive plaques	Supraoptic paraventric. nuclei	Median eminence	Corticospinal tracts
Natural Scrapie 34 cases	+ (2 cases)	+	+	−	Preserved	No demyelination	Degenerated	*	+ (4 cases)	Degenerated	Excess of NS material	Normal
Kuru 13 cases	+ (1 case)	+	+	+ (7 cases) in limited parts of cortex and in striatum	Preserved (except in spongy areas)	No demyelination	Very severe degeneration	Moderate degeneration	+ (except 3 cases)	Normal	Excess of NS material	Degenerated (6 out of 12 cases)
Exp. Kuru 15 cases	+ (2 cases)	−	+	Severe throughout	Destroyed throughout	No demyelination	Moderate degeneration	Slight degeneration	?	Normal	Excess of NS material	Normal
Polioencephalopathy 2 cases	−	−	+	Severe throughout	Destroyed throughout	No demyelination	Very severe degeneration	Very severe degeneration	−	Moderate degeneration	Empty of NS material	Normal (+ in lit.)

* = The neo-cerebellar component in the sheep is very small.
(+ in Lit.) = Some cases of subacute presenile polioencephalopathy with degeneration of the cortico-spinal tracts are recorded in the literature.

there was some generalized fibrous gliosis, somewhat more severe in the olives. The striatum and some of the thalamic nuclei were degenerated and there was nerve cell loss in the supraoptic and paraventricular nuclei of the hypothalamus. The cerebral cortex was atrophic, and in many regions reduced to about half its normal width. Here there was status spongiosus (Fig. 26D) with great neuronal loss, proliferation of fibrous and gemistocytic astrocytes (Fig. 25D) and of microglial cells, leading to complete obliteration of the cortical architecture. In many areas these changes were so severe that 'sponginess' was no longer obvious owing to an apparent collapse of the tissue. At the time of biopsy, five months before the patient's death, the cortex was better preserved, although status spongiosus was already well developed.

Experimentally induced subacute presenile polioencephalopathy
Examination of the chimpanzee's brain, A54, which had been inoculated with material from the above case (Gibbs *et al.* 1968) was conducted in parallel on coded specimens from a neurologically normal animal and an animal with experimental Kuru. The changes in A54 were sufficiently distinct to permit a blind differential diagnosis. The full investigation has not yet been completed, but preliminary studies show that there was status spongiosus of the cerebral cortex with intense proliferation of astrocytes but also of microglial cells; this is one of the distinguishing features from experimental Kuru where, as a rule, the cortex does not contain active microglial cells. There was further a considerable loss of Betz' giant cells in the motor cortex, these cells being remarkably well preserved in Kuru but often affected in polioencephalopathy. Lastly there were unusual large neurones with pale cytoplasm, often containing an ill-defined inclusion. Similar cells were found in the brain of the patient with polioencephalopathy. The cerebellum of A54 showed only moderate degeneration, as did the brainstem, although the pontine nuclei were severely affected.

Comment
In Table 11 Scrapie, Kuru, experimental Kuru and subacute presenile polioencephalopathy are arranged according to similarities and differences in the pattern of their principal neuropathological changes. Clinically they are all subacute degenerations of the brain, usually presenting with ataxia. They are relentlessly progressive and, on average, fatal within a few months; none of them appear to be contagious, but all can be transmitted to experimental animals. On the pathological

side there are also great similarities, for all these diseases cause a primary degeneration of the grey matter with a severe astrocytic reaction, but with only secondary involvement of the white matter; degeneration of the cerebellar and the hypothalamo-neurohypophysial system is seen in all and none show consistently any features which could be interpreted as an inflammatory reaction. Last, but not least, status spongiosus of the grey matter features in natural Kuru and in polioencephalopathy as well as in all the experimentally induced conditions including experimental Scrapie. On the other hand there are a number of differences. Thus the occurrence of coarsely vacuolated neurones is restricted to Scrapie and Kuru. Such vacuolation was seen neither in experimental Kuru nor in polioencephalopathy, either in our own cases or in those reported in the literature; further, the cortical architecture is preserved in Scrapie and, to a great extent, in Kuru, while it is obliterated in experimental Kuru and in our own cases of polioencephalopathy, though cases with better preservation are on record; cerebellar degeneration which is uniform throughout in polioencephalopathy, is in Kuru more severe in the paleocerebellar structures; PAS positive plaques are only found in Scrapie and in Kuru and lastly the cortico-spinal tracts remain normal in Scrapie and experimental Kuru.

ACKNOWLEDGEMENT

We should like to acknowledge support from The Research Fund of the Bethlem Royal and Maudsley Hospitals and the Nuffield Foundation.

REFERENCES

BECK E., DANIEL P. M. & PARRY H. B. (1964) Degeneration of the cerebellar and hypothalamo-neurohypophysial systems in sheep with Scrapie; and its relationship to human system degenerations. *Brain*, **87**, 153–176.

BECK E. & DANIEL P. M. (1965a) Kuru and Scrapie compared: are they examples of system degeneration? In: *Slow, Latent and Temperate Virus Infections*. National Institute of Neurological Diseases and Blindness. Monograph No. 2, pp. 85–93. U.S. Department of Health, Education and Welfare.

BECK E. & DANIEL P. M. (1965b) Observations on the pathology of experimentally produced Scrapie. In: *Slow, Latent and Temperate Virus Infections*. National Institute of Neurological Diseases and Blindness. Monograph No. 2, pp. 203–206 U.S. Department of Health, Education and Welfare.

BECK E., DANIEL P. M. & GAJDUSEK D. C. (1966) A comparison between the neuropathological changes in Kuru and in Scrapie. A system degeneration. *Int. Congr. Neuropath.* pp. 213–218. Excerpta Med. International Congress Series No. 100.

BECK E., DANIEL P.M., ALPERS M., GAJDUSEK D.C. & GIBBS C.J. JR (1966) Experimental 'Kuru' in chimpanzees. A pathological report. *Lancet* ii, 1056–1059.

BERTRAND I., CARRÉ H. & LUCAM F. (1937) La 'tremblante' du mouton. *Ann. Anat. path.*, **14**, 565–586.

BROWNELL B. & OPPENHEIMER D.R. (1965) An ataxic form of subacute presenile polioencephalopathy (Creutzfeldt-Jakob disease). *J. Neurol. Neurosurg. Psychiat.* **28**, 350–361.

FOWLER M. & ROBERTSON E.G. (1959) Observations on Kuru. III Pathological features in five cases. *Australasian Ann. Med.* **8**, 16–26.

GIBBS C.J. JR, GAJDUSEK D.C., ASHER D.M., ALPERS M.P., BECK E., DANIEL P.M. & MATTHEWS W.B. (1968) Creutzfeldt-Jakob disease (spongiform encephalopathy): Transmission to the chimpanzee. *Science*, **161**, 388–389.

HADLOW W.J. (1959) Scrapie and Kuru. *Lancet*, ii, 289–290.

HADLOW W.J. (1961) The pathology of experimental Scrapie in the dairy goat. *Res. Vet. Sci.* **2**, 289–314.

JONES D.P. & NEVIN S. (1954). Rapidly progressive cerebral degeneration (subacute vascular encephalopathy) with mental disorder, focal disturbances and myoclonic epilepsy. *J. Neurol. Neurosurg. Psychiat.* **17**, 148–159.

KAKULAS B.A., LECOURS A.R. & GAJDUSEK D.C. (1967) Further observations on the pathology of Kuru. A study of the two cerebra in serial sections. *J. Neuropath. exp. Neurol.* **26**, 85–97.

KLATZO I., GAJDUSEK D.C. & ZIGAS V. (1959) Pathology of Kuru. *Lab. Invest.* **8**, 799–847.

NEVIN S., MCMENEMEY W.H., BEHRMAN S. & JONES D.P. (1960) Subacute spongiform encephalopathy—a subacute form of encephalopathy attributable to vascular dysfunction (Spongiform cerebral atrophy). *Brain*, **83**, 519–564.

NEUMANN M.A., GAJDUSEK D.C. & ZIGAS V. (1964) Neuropathologic findings in exotic neurologic disorders among natives of the highlands of New Guinea. *J. Neuropath. exp. Neurol.* **23**, 486–507.

PATTISON I.H. & SMITH K. (1963) Histological observations on experimental Scrapie in the mouse. *Res. Vet. Sci.* **4**, 269–275.

PATTISON I.H. (1965) Experiments with Scrapie with special reference to the nature of the agent and the pathology of the disease. In: *Slow, Latent and Temperate Virus Infections.* National Institute of Neurological Diseases and Blindness. Monograph No. 2, pp. 249–255. U.S. Department of Health, Education and Welfare.

SHIRAKI H. (1966) Closing remarks by the Chairman. *Int. Congr. Neuropath.* pp. 222–224. Excerpta Med. International Congress Series No. 100.

ZIGAS V. & GAJDUSEK D.C. (1957) Kuru: clinical study of a new syndrome resembling paralysis agitans in natives of the eastern highlands of Australian New Guinea. *Med. J. Austr.*, **2**, 745–754.

The Clinical Details of the Case of Subacute Presenile Polio-encephalopathy Discussed by Mrs Beck

W. B. Matthews

The patient, a man of 59, was admitted to the Derbyshire Royal Infirmary eight weeks after the abrupt onset of visual disturbance, initially micropsia. Mental confusion developed rapidly and on admission he was already helpless, lying with the upper limbs rigid in flexion and the lower limbs in extension. He was conscious and responsive to stimuli but speech was limited to an occasional monosyllable. Myoclonus was inconspicuous at that time but soon became a prominent feature involving all limbs and the head, although showing great variation in distribution and severity. Deterioration continued and he became mute and unresponsive with all limbs in rigid flexion.

The EEG showed periodic high voltage stereotyped spike discharges. The CSF protein was slightly raised being 80 and 60 mg/100 ml on the two occasions it was examined.

He died five months from the onset of his illness.

The Chemical Nature of the Scrapie Agent

G. D. Hunter

Until recently, most workers in the field considered that the Scrapie agent was likely to be closely related to conventional viruses (Stamp 1962, Hunter 1965) and this view is still held by many people (e.g. Eklund, Hadlow & Kennedy 1967, Adams & Caspary 1967). However, as long as eight years ago, Palmer (1960) suggested that the Scrapie agent might be composed at least partially of carbohydrate and some arguments against the viral hypothesis have been reiterated more recently by Pattison (1965).

Attempts to release a viral-type agent from Scrapie-affected brain have not been successful, although extensive experimentation has been carried out with this aim in view (Hunter & Millson 1967, Mould, private communication). Similarly, efforts to visualize the Scrapie agent electron microscopically have given essentially negative results (Chandler 1968, Field & Raine 1964). No marked changes from the normal situation have been noted in the patterns of RNA and protein bio-synthesis in Scrapie brain (Kimberlin 1968, Millson & Hunter 1968). An increased rate of DNA synthesis has been detected in Scrapie brain (Kimberlin & Hunter 1967), but the newly synthesized DNA is con-fined to the cell nucleus, whereas the Scrapie agent is mainly located in the cytoplasmic organelles (Hunter, Millson & Meek 1964, Kimberlin & Hunter 1967, Kimberlin, unpublished work). It has also been shown autoradiographically (Kimberlin & Anger 1968) that the number of active brain nuclei reaches a maximum three to six weeks after inocula-tion of Scrapie material intracerebrally (Fig. 28), long before there is any appreciable accumulation of the Scrapie agent in affected brain.

Purely virological investigations have also failed to provide much support for the viral hypothesis in Scrapie, but negative evidence is of limited value. Substantial positive evidence against the viral hypothesis was, however, forthcoming when Alper, Haig & Clarke (1966) showed that the Scrapie agent was completely resistant to the action of ultra-violet light in the wavelength range where nucleic acids absorb maxi-mally. It is very difficult, although not completely impossible (Gibbons & Hunter 1967) to reconcile these results with an appreciable informational nucleic acid content for the Scrapie agent. The inactivation of the Scrapie agent with ionizing radiation (Alper *et al.* 1966) also indicated a rather improbably small size for a viral agent. In addition, further studies by Alper, Cramp, Haig & Clarke (1967) have shown that the Scrapie agent is insensitive to ultraviolet light in the region where most proteins are absorbent.

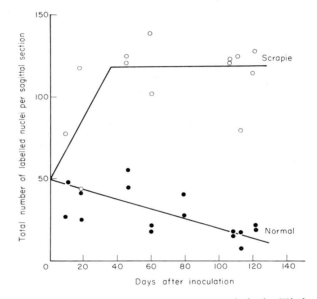

FIGURE 28. Labelled nuclei in normal and Scrapie brain (Kimberlin & Anger 1968). ○ Scrapie nuclei   ● normal nuclei.

With the foregoing results in mind, the possibility that the agent might contain a substantial and important polysaccharide component was investigated in the Biochemistry Dept. at Compton. There was on the biochemical side already some evidence to suggest that Scrapie-affected brain might be responding to the presence of foreign carbohydrate (Millson 1965, Hunter & Millson 1966, Hunter, Millson & Vockins 1967, Mackenzie, Millson & Wilson 1968): increased activity of glyco- sidase enzymes is a prominent feature in the development of Scrapie disease. The outcome of these experimental investigations was interest- ing and largely unexpected. One finding did suggest that the agent might contain an important polysaccharide component. Scrapie activity was rapidly destroyed by the action of o·o1 M periodate under conditions where the destruction of protein and nucleic acid would be minimal but polysaccharide would be specifically attacked (Fig. 29, Hunter, Millson & Gibbons 1967, Hunter, Gibbons, Kimberlin & Millson 1968). Nevertheless, strong urea solutions and aqueous phenol, reagents widely used for the extraction in intact form of polysaccharides, were found to destroy the agent (Hunter *et al.* 1968, Mould, private communication).

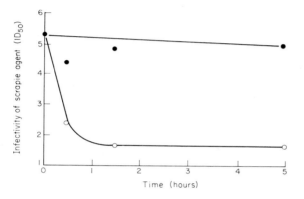

FIGURE 29. Inactivation of the Scrapie agent with o·o1 M periodate, pH 3·5 (Hunter, Gibbons, Kimberlin & Millson 1968). ○ periodate treatment ● iodate-treated controls.

These findings, taken together with other information about the Scrapie agent (Table 12), led to a puzzling situation. There was strong evidence against it being identified with any of the known major groups of simple macromolecules (Gibbons & Hunter 1967). Most of the results could, however, be explained in terms of the existence of an infective molecular complex containing protein, polysaccharide and perhaps lipid also. A re-examination of earlier work involving cellular fractionation showed clearly that all fractions rich in cellular membrane possessed high Scrapie titres (Hunter *et al.* 1964, Mould, Smith & Dawson 1965), and the most likely location of such a complex seemed to be as part of such a structure. The membrane hypothesis proposed by Gibbons & Hunter (1967) made essentially three statements: (1) the Scrapie agent is an integral part of a membrane structure in or around affected cells; (2) the alteration in affected cell membranes may largely involve polysaccharide molecules; (3) replication may proceed by an

TABLE 12. Stability of the Scrapie agent in various physical and chemical situations

Treatment	Effect
Ionizing radiation	$D_0 = 4\cdot3$ Mrads
Ultraviolet radiation at 240, 254, 265, 280, 290, 315 and 330 mμ	Negligible loss of titre with incident doses up to 5×10^4 ergs/mm^2.
Heat at 100°C for 10–60 min	Substantial, but incomplete loss of titre
Heat at 80°C for 60 min	Negligible loss of titre
Treatment with fluorocarbon at 0°–4°C	Negligible loss of titre
Heat at 80°C for 20 min after fluorocarbon treatment	Substantial loss of titre
Treatment with ether at room temperature	Partial loss of titre
Acid and alkali	Essentially stable in pH range 2·5–10·5. Destroyed by strong acid and alkali
Formalin, 0·5–18%	Highly resistant. Some loss of titre but no accurate quantitative data available
β-Propionolactone, 1%	Slight loss of titre
0·01 molar periodate at pH 4 at room temperature	Substantial loss of titre
6 molar or 8 molar urea	Substantial or complete loss of titre
90% phenol	Substantial or complete loss of titre
Strong salt solutions (for example, 6 molar lithium chloride, caesium chloride and ammonium sulphate)	Titre readily lost under various conditions
Detergents	Relatively stable in the presence of neutral detergents and 0·01 molar sodium deoxycholate
Proteolytic enzymes	Partial loss of titre after fluorocarbon treatment, but very little before it
DNase, RNase, lipase, phospholipase a, phospholipase c, neuraminidase, β-glucuronidase	No effect on titre of crude preparations

extension of known processes leading to the production of polysaccharides. The third statement was rather general in its nature, and a more convincing model for the replication of a Scrapie-affected membrane may perhaps be made by applying the theory of 'membrane constraint' (Changeux, Thiéry, Tung & Kittel 1967) to the Scrapie situation (Hunter, Kimberlin & Gibbons 1968). It is possible that there is no difference at all in chemical composition between normal and Scrapie-affected membranes, merely a change in the physical conformation of membrane sub-units.

A decision between the viral and membrane hypotheses for Scrapie must await the outcome of further work; and it is highly probable that whatever hypothesis eventually proves to be nearest to the truth will require considerable modification and elaboration from present forms.

REFERENCES

ADAMS D.H. & CASPARY E.A. (1967) Nature of the Scrapie virus. *Brit. med. J.* iii, 173.

ALPER T., CRAMP W.A., HAIG D.A. & CLARKE M.C. (1967) Does the agent of Scrapie replicate without nucleic acid? *Nature, Lond.* **214**, 764–766.

ALPER T., HAIG D.A. & CLARKE M.C. (1966) The exceptionally small size of the Scrapie agent. *Biochem. biophys. Res. Commun.* **22**, 278–284.

CHANDLER R.L. (1968) Ultrastructural pathology of Scrapie in the mouse: an electron microscopic study of spinal cord and cerebellar areas. *Br. J. exp. Path.* **49**, 52–59.

CHANGEUX J.P., THIÉRY J., TUNG Y. & KITTEL C. (1967) On the cooperativity of biological membranes. *Proc. Natl. Acad. Sci.* **57**, 335–341.

EKLUND C.M., KENNEDY R.C. & HADLOW W.J. (1967) Pathogenesis of Scrapie virus infection in the mouse. *J. Inf. Diseases*, **117**, 15–22.

FIELD E.J. & RAINE C.S. (1964) An electron microscopic study of Scrapie in the mouse. *Acta Neuropath.* **4**, 200–211.

GIBBONS R.A. & HUNTER G.D. (1967) Nature of the Scrapie agent. *Nature, Lond.* **215**, 1041–1043.

HUNTER G.D. (1965) Progress towards the isolation and characterization of the Scrapie agent. *Nat. Inst. Nervous Diseases and Blindness Monograph No.* 2. pp. 259–262.

HUNTER G.D., GIBBONS R.A., KIMBERLIN R.H. & MILLSON G.C. (1968) Further studies of the infectivity and stability of extracts and homogenates derived from Scrapie affected mouse brains. *J. comp. Path.* **20**, 355–357.

HUNTER G.D., KIMBERLIN, R.H. & GIBBONS R.A. (1968) Scrapie: a modified membrane hypothesis. *J. theoret. Biol.* in the press.

HUNTER G.D. & MILLSON G.C. (1966) Distribution and activation of lysosomal enzyme activities in subcellular components of normal and Scrapie-affected mouse brain. *J. Neurochem.* **13**, 375–383.

HUNTER G.D., MILLSON G.C. & GIBBONS R.A. (1967) Some new information concerning the stability of the Scrapie agent. *Biochem. J.* **105**, 7P.

HUNTER G.D., MILLSON G.C. & MEEK G. (1964) The intracellular location of the agent of mouse Scrapie. *J. gen. Microbiol.* **34**, 319–325.

HUNTER G.D., MILLSON G.C. & VOCKINS M.D. (1967) Lysosomal enzymes and Scrapie. *Biochem. J.* **102**, 43P.

KIMBERLIN R.H. (1968) RNA metabolism in the brains of mice clinically affected with Scrapie. *J. comp. Path.* **78**, 237.

KIMBERLIN R.H. & ANGER H.S. (1968) DNA synthesis in the glial cells of Scrapie-affected mouse brain. *J. Neurochem.* In the press.

KIMBERLIN R.H. & HUNTER G.D. (1967) DNA synthesis in Scrapie-affected mouse brain. *J. gen. Virology*, **1**, 115–124.

MACKENZIE A., MILLSON G.C. & WILSON A.M. (1968) Glycosidase histochemistry in normal and Scrapie mice, rats, sheep and goats. *J. comp. Path.* **78**, 43–52.

MILLSON G.C. (1965) Lysosomal enzymes in normal and Scrapie mouse brain. *J. Neurochem.* **12**, 461–468.

MILLSON G.C. & HUNTER G.D. (1968) Protein synthesis in normal and Scrapie mouse brain. *J. Neurochem.* **15**, 447–453.

MOULD D.L., SMITH W. & DAWSON A.McL. (1965) Centrifugation studies on the infectivities of cellular fractions derived from mouse brain infected with Scrapie ('Suffolk'). *J. gen. Microbiol.* **40**, 71–79.

PALMER A.C. (1960) *Progress in the biological sciences in relation to dermatology*, p. 239, Cambridge.

PATTISON I.H. (1965) Resistance of the Scrapie agent to formalin. *J. comp. Path.* **75**, 159–164.

STAMP J.T. (1962) Scrapie: a transmissible disease of sheep. *Vet. Rec.* **74**, 357.

The Virology of Scrapie

D. A. Haig

The causal agent of Scrapie has not yet been characterized and there have been numerous speculations concerning its nature. Nevertheless, it is apparent that this agent is transmissible in series and that it is filterable. For these reasons it is usually classed as a virus, as it is in Andrewes' recent book. However, there is an accumulating amount of evidence to show that the agent of Scrapie has many unusual properties for a virus and this has led a number of workers to doubt the validity of this classification (see Pattison 1965). The more remarkable of the points about the agent and the disease properties are its great heat stability and resistance to formalin, lack of any demonstrable antibody response and the markedly bilateral symmetry of the pathological changes which consist of degeneration without any sign of an inflammatory response. It has not been cultivated *in vitro*, nor has it been seen under the electron microscope.

The natural disease has long been thought to be genetic in origin and there is no doubt that genetic factors govern susceptibility and length of incubation period. Experimentally the disease has been transmitted not only from sheep to sheep but also to the goat, mouse, rat and hamster. It was the finding of Chandler in 1961 that the mouse is susceptible to the experimental disease which made quantitative work on Scrapie possible and has helped speed up the work. Transmission is possible by almost any route including oral dosing, and it is perhaps by this route that the disease is transmitted in nature, contact infections under experimental conditions having been reported, although the mechanism is unknown. This would support the virus theory.

In affected animals greatest activity of the agent is found in the CNS but it is present to fairly high titre in other organs such as the spleen, lymph nodes and various glands. Traces have been found in the blood of mice but it is not certain whether these are due to contamination with tissue during the collection of the sample. Field (1967) has shown that following peripheral inoculation the earliest Scrapie reaction is found in the corresponding segments of the neuraxis, suggesting an early blood dissemination of the agent and he has likened the pathogenesis of Scrapie to that of 'a good old fashioned neurotropic virus'. Eklund, Kennedy & Hadlow (1967) have shown that following subcutaneous injection the agent rapidly increases in quantity in the spleen and only later invades the brain. This, they too, have likened to known viral findings.

In any consideration of the nature of a transmissible agent, particle size is of major importance. Since the agent of Scrapie has not yet been freed from tissue debris to which it appears to be firmly bound there are technical difficulties connected with filtration experiments. The agent will pass readily through membranes of 210 mμ APD and there is an unconfirmed report of a successful filtration by Gibbs (1967) through a membrane of 43 mμ giving a calculated size of 26 mμ, well within the known virus range. On the other hand, exposure to ionizing irradiation of freeze-dried preparations sealed under oxygen gave a Do value as high as 4·3 mrads with a molecular weight of about 1·5 × 10^5. From this a target size of about 7 mμ was calculated (Alper, Cramp, Haig & Clarke 1967). If this were nucleic acid it could code only for a maximum of about 150 amino acids. This makes it unlikely that the agent has a thick protein coat such as has been postulated would be necessary to protect it from damage by chemical and physical treatments. Because this size seemed improbably small for a virus we then studied the effect of irradiation with ultraviolet light of various wavelengths. It was found that large doses of ultraviolet irradiation at 254 mμ, a wavelength specifically absorbed by nucleic acid, had no apparent effect on the activity of the agent. While the significance of these findings is debatable, one possibility which must be considered is that the agent is able to replicate without itself containing NA. Our irradiation results have, I believe, been confirmed by other workers, but they disagree with our conclusions and they feel that the agent could be a virus containing perhaps a small nucleic acid core with possibly a carbohydrate coat (Adams & Caspary 1967).

It has also been claimed that alkylating agents such as β-propiolactone have a marked depressing effect on the activity of all viruses against which they have been tested. We have noted that although BPL does reduce infectivity of the Scrapie agent this is considerably less than for known viruses and is roughly similar to that of ether, indicating perhaps that the damage done by BPL is not due to its action on nucleic acid or protein but that some other component is involved.

Until such time as the Scrapie agent is isolated in pure form conjecture on its nature will continue, but I feel one is justified in doubting its classification as a virus.

REFERENCES

ADAMS D.H. & CASPARY E.A. (1967) Nature of the Scrapie virus. *Brit. med. J.* iii, 173–174.

ALPER T., CRAMP W.A., HAIG D.A. & CLARKE M.C. (1967) Does the Scrapie agent replicate without nucleic acid? *Nature*, **214**, 764–766.

CHANDLER R.L. (1961) Encephalopathy in mice by inoculation of Scrapie brain material. *Lancet*, i, 1378–1380.

EKLUND C.M., KENNEDY R.C. & HADLOW W.J. (1967) Pathogenesis of Scrapie virus in the mouse. *J. inf. Dis.* **117**, 15–22.

FIELD E.J. (1967) Invasion of the mouse nervous system by Scrapie. *Br. J. exp. Path.* **48**, 662–664.

GIBBS C.J. (1967) *Current Topics in Microbiology*. **40**, 44. Berlin.

PATTISON I.H. (1965) Resistance of the Scrapie agent to formalin. *J. Comp. Path.* **75**, 159–164.

Virus and Provirus in the Evolution of Disease

C. D. Darlington

The distinction between heredity and infection, which at first seemed too simple to define, has now become the most complex problem in the study of disease. It is also a practical problem whenever diseases of obscure origin are being discussed. The difficulty began with the discovery of the Rous sarcoma in 1910. It was made worse when much later DNA and RNA were found to be equally necessary for each type of genetic particle, hereditary or infectious. But it was made easier when such particles were found to have the same possibilities of genetic permanence in the cytoplasm that they had in the nucleus (Darlington 1939, 1944). The history of transmission rather than chemical or structural character seemed then to become the effective criterion; for this reason I proposed the term *provirus* to distinguish two kinds of selective and evolutionary history.

In introducing this term I defined the provirus as a genetic particle having all the properties of a virus in experiment save that of natural infection. It could be responsible for neoplastic tumours in animals or plants; as such it could be generated or released by irradiation and by chemical treatment or by infection with unrelated organisms; and it could arise in or attach itself to, plants, animals and bacteria (Darlington & Mather 1949, Darlington 1948, 1949a, b, 1960).

These attempts at definition have been justified by the adoption of the term, whether correctly or incorrectly, by its present convenience, and by the experimental evidence of the origin of viruses. At the same time the opinion underlying the definition has been strengthened by experience. Selection by heredity and selection by infection do in fact seem to be two divergent evolutionary pathways having a common origin whether close at hand or utterly remote.

It now appears however that not one but at least three situations may place a particle in the category of provirus.

First, there is the free and freely diffusible particle of RNA or DNA which has no organization to distinguish it from any other stable or self-propagating hereditary cell constituent. Such a particle is a plasmagene. It is also a provirus *sensu stricto*.

133

Secondly, there is the hereditary particle whose elaborate structure and unique properties point to an ancient infectious ancestry. Such is Sonneborn's Kappa particle in *Paramecium*.

Thirdly, there are all the latent viruses of insects whose organization implies an ancestry which has long been optional or alternative, either infectious or hereditary (Longworth & Cunningham 1968). Here also are the genetic precursors of the infectious bacteriophages to which Lwoff gave the name of pro-phages.

These three classes all contribute to showing us that genetic particles may pass over from heredity to infection and *vice versa*; and that they do so both in the life of the individual and in the evolution of the species.

But it is the first class of strict proviruses which matter to us in connection with the kinds of disputed cases we are dealing with today.

The strict proviruses stretch from the leukaemia agents in mice (Darlington 1959) to the artificially infectious plasmagenes which are natural in some plants (Frankel 1962), although chemically or bacterially induced in others (Darlington 1949b). The classical instance however is the agent of the Rous sarcoma. This tumour could at first be transferred only to a fowl of the inbred strain in which it arose. But later by mutation and selection it evidently became adaptable and could be used to infect other breeds and even other species. But it will remain a strictly artificial virus unless or until, by changes in both heredity and environment, it finds some other vector than the human experimenter.

The Rous sarcoma provirus is a particle having no conceivable infectious history yet it has been converted to unbalanced propagation and hence to a potential virus character. Just this conversion, we now know, can happen not only in the spontaneous origin of fowl tumours but also in the generation of leukaemia in mice by irradiation (Lieberman & Kaplan 1959). Which in turn is what we should expect from the generation of infectious tumours in plants (Darlington 1949b).

Such evolutionary changes are, however, well known in proviruses. The Shope papilloma virus changes its mode of activity and transmission when it is transferred from a cottontail to a European rabbit. And the Bittner agent which could not be transmitted naturally if it affected a bird, is transmitted naturally through the milk of a mammal. Similarly leukaemia which cannot be passed artificially between adult mice can be passed between day-old mice. Such experience suggests what practical steps are needed for evolution from an hereditary to an infectious way of life.

There is therefore a distinction, a practical distinction, between an artificially infective pro-virus and the naturally infective true virus to which it may so easily give rise.

A variety of circumstances, due to differences between species of host, or to environmental or developmental differences such as mode of feeding or age, lead in fact to the transformation of an hereditary into an infectious particle; and also of an artificially into a naturally infectious particle. This is evolution in one direction and it is characteristic of our strict class of proviruses. But of evolution in the reverse direction the other two classes provide the evidence. The Kappa particles in *Paramecium* are assumed to have an infectious ancestry, the means of infection being now limited to copulation; but they are now integrated both in the physiological life of the individual and also in the genetic system of the species.

When we consider insect viruses from this point of view we find that what was a source of ambiguity becomes a means of understanding. The *Rickettsia* virus, or super-virus, may pass indefinitely through the egg of the bug which carries it. The same transmission is believed to hold for the polyhedroses of insects in general (Smith 1958). From the point of view of the virologist such viruses are said to be *latent*. Their structure, so highly adapted for infection, leaves little doubt that they have an evolutionary history as natural viruses. They are not true proviruses or beginners. But from the point of view of long-term evolution itself we are bound to notice that the virus is, in the case of *Rickettsia*, part of the genetic system of the insect and depends for its survival on some benefit it confers on the stocks with which it co-exists. And if the human victim were to disappear the virus would continue as an unconditional and unambiguous hereditary particle.

Which course one of the momentarily ambiguous agents may take has been shown to depend on both hereditary and environmental variables. In the moth *Abraxas grossulariata*, inbreeding can expose the recessive polymorphic variety *lacticolor* which has the specific property of activating a latent virus capable of infecting and killing the normal moths. This is an elaborately adapted virus which dons a protein coat but has existed in the normal species, we must suppose, as an RNA component of one of its cytoplasmic organellae. Similar generation of a virus by various treatments in the silkworm *Bombyx mori* is likewise restricted to specific genotypes (Yamafuji *et al.* 1961).

With such diverse evolutionary possibilities new viruses are continually being created. Some are created by experimental transplantation from one species to another (Smith 1952). In nature however insects must make such experiments on a far larger scale. Most new viruses no doubt disappear quickly. A few explode in brief epidemics. Those that are known best to virologists are bound for the most part to be the ones in which the propagation of host and parasite are successfully and lastingly balanced. It is in the light of this experience and these expectations that we have to look for the causes of Kuru and Scrapie.

The most probable explanation of both these diseases seems to be that each is the result of the action of a homozygous recessive gene which slowly affects the generation of self-replicating RNA particles in the nerve cells. These particles cannot be transmitted by normal processes of infection or contagion in the case of either disease. But in the case of Kuru they have been transmitted to a high proportion of the kindred in inbred stocks of the Fore tribes of central New Guinea. These tribes practise the eating of kindred, that is of friends rather than enemies (Glasse 1967, Gajdusek 1967). This is an unusual type of cannibalism and it is the most dangerous that could be conceived for giving a highly host-specific disease its opportunity. But since the women were most addicted to this consumption of flesh the sex ratio of the tribe was upset and women were imported. The heterogeneity of the tribe created in this way, together with the decline of cannibalism, no doubt diminished the impact of Kuru. The whole cycle has been completed in two or three generations.

With Scrapie, on the other hand, there is no evidence of natural infection. There is evidence, however, of artificial selection. The disease has expanded, on the evidence of the records, through selection for rapid maturity, selection operating on heterozygotes. The recessive gene appears to have been favoured through the maintenance of the balanced polymorphism that has resulted from this selection over a period of a few hundred generations (Parry 1962, Draper 1963). On this view Scrapie is genetically and physiologically analogous with a much discussed disease of a plant which has been similarly subjected to a high pressure of artificial selection for productivity. This is the Yellows disease of cultivated strawberry varieties, breakdown occurring in strawberries after many years of cultivation. It is degenerative or abiotrophic. It is genetically controlled and hereditary. It is not infectious but in symptoms it resembles a virus disease (Darlington & Mather, 1949).

In the situations of Kuru and Scrapie (and also strawberry yellows) we have to suppose that messenger RNA derived from particular genes cumulatively affects the character of stable RNA particles in the cytoplasm of particular tissues so as to damage the activity of the cells. And the modified particles or the modifying agents are transmissible by artificial inoculation although not by natural infection. Except so far as, in the case of Kuru, we regard kindred-cannibalism as a natural mode of life.

Summing up

To study evolution in viruses we have to compare their transmission and modification in plants and protista, in arthropods and vertebrates, and in bacteria. We also have to examine their relations with each of the hosts, the victim or the vector as examples of adaptation either to infection or heredity. And we have to pay special attention to modes of origin and transmission of agents used in the causation of cancer in birds and mammals, insects and plants.

The experimental evidence indicates that normally hereditary particles may give rise to artificially infectious particles or proviruses from which in turn naturally infectious viruses may appear. Beyond this hereditary or latent particles may become infective particles and *vice versa*. The transformation may occur reversibly between successive generations. And it may also occur not reversibly on an evolutionary scale.

For this, it may be activated by the direct agency of specific nucleic acids or collaterally, as we may say, by related proteins or polysaccharides; or again by shifts in external conditions or in habits of feeding.

The causation of diseases such as Kuru and Scrapie having combined genetic, cytoplasmic and pro-viral components must be examined in the light of these selective and evolutionary connections and is likely to throw its own light on the origins and behaviour of viruses in general.

REFERENCES

DARLINGTON C.D. (1939) *Evolution of Genetic Systems.* Cambridge.
DARLINGTON C.D. (1958) *Evolution of Genetic Systems.* (2nd ed.), Edinburgh.
DARLINGTON C.D. (1944) Heredity, development and infection. *Nature*, **154**, 164–169.
DARLINGTON C.D. (1949a) The working units of heredity. *Hereditas* (Suppl. Vol.).
DARLINGTON C.D. (1949b) Les Plasmagènes. In: *Unités biologiques douées de continuité génétique*, pp. 123–130.
DARLINGTON C.D. (1959) Plasmagene theory and cancer genesis. In: *Genetics and Cancer*, Texas.

DARLINGTON C.D. (1960) Origin and evolution of viruses. *Trans. R.S. Trop. Med. and Hygiene*, **54**, 90–96.

DARLINGTON C.D. & MATHER K. (1949) *The Elements of Genetics*. London.

DRAPER G.J. (1963) 'Epidemics' caused by a late-manifesting gene. Application to Scrapie. *Heredity*, **18**, 165–171.

FRANKEL R. (1962) Further evidence on graft induced transmission to progeny of cytoplasmic male sterility in Petunia. *Genetics*, **47**, 641–646.

GLASSE R. (1967) Cannibalism in the Kuru region of New Guinea. *Trans. New York Acad. Sci.* **29**, 748–754.

GAJDUSEK, D.C. (1967) Slow-virus infections of the nervous system. *New England Journ. Med.* **276**, 392–400.

LIEBERMAN M. & KAPLAN H.S. (1959) Leukemogenic activity of filtrates from radiation-induced lymphoid tumours of mice. *Science*, **130**, 387–388.

LONGWORTH J.F. & CUNNINGHAM J.C. (1968) The activation of occult nuclear-polyhedrosis viruses by foreign nuclear polyhedra. *J. Invert. Path*, **10** (in the press).

PARRY H.B. (1962) A transmissible and hereditary disease of sheep. *Heredity*, **17**, 75–105.

SMITH K.M. (1952) Latency in viruses and the production of new virus diseases. *Biol. Reviews*, **27**, 347–357.

SMITH K.M. & WILLIAMS R.C. (1958) Insect viruses and their structure. *Endeavour*, **17**, 12–21.

YAMAFUJI, K. & YOSHIHARA F. (1961) A gene synthesizing protease and a pre-viral genome in silkworms. *Nature*, **192**, 782.

Discussion on Kuru and Scrapie

McMenemy: I would like to start by asking Dr Alpers a little practical point of gastronomy. Do these people who get Kuru eat the brains or do they eat the body in general, and also do they cook or do they eat them raw?

Alpers: They eat the whole body even including the faeces and there are certain parts of the body which are reserved for certain privileged kinsfolk. The offal, as with the pig, will usually go to the women and children, so it's the women and children mainly who eat the brain. Men eat the well cooked selected pieces of meat and this is a normal pattern of a feast. However cooking is very limited and in many cases the selected parts are taken away and incubated in the huts for a few days before they are consumed, so all kinds of things may have got in at the same time.

Hunter: I think it is only fair to point out that there have been other groups which made extensive studies of natural scrapie in the field and have a different interpretation of Dr Parry's own results. If we confine ourselves merely to Dickinson's and Stamp's studies, they appear to have fairly convincing evidence for a general and not a complex genetic control of susceptibility and maternal transmission of the agent. May I ask Dr Parry, in view of the fact that contagious infection can occur in Scrapie—transfer of this natural disease by contact from sheep to the goat is known, as well as the experiment that Dr Haig mentioned—and in view of the fact that we know the agent can certainly be passed by overgrazing, does he think that perhaps both groups might be right? Might contagious transfer be more important in the flocks that Dickinson & Stamp have studied which may differ from his?

Parry: This is entirely possible although the group in Edinburgh have not got the data on natural flocks. They have data on information from the laboratory devised under their conditions. They have not got the data on a natural population under accurate control with accurately supervised records, as far as I know. A number of sheep they used on which their view was based came from flocks of which I know something. I do not accept that they were told the whole truth about the animals with which they were working. I have been misled often enough myself, and this also applies to the comment that Dr Haig made about contact spread to a group of Scottish hill sheep called Scotch Blackface. We had exactly the same story 10 years ago with Welsh mountain sheep which were alleged not to have Scrapie and therefore could be assumed to have contracted it by contact. We know now that the disease is widespread and of a genetic character in this breed. The position is exactly the same in the Scottish Blackface. To get at the truth of the matter, either in Wales or in Scotland, is more difficult than in New Guinea!

WEBB: May I ask Dr Alpers and Dr Hunter, in a very early case of Scrapie or Kuru do you see astrocytosis? Because if so we must come back to the possibility of an agent which can transform cells, and which can be transmitted by a cell line. This point of view might suggest a newer way of investigating a number of diseases in which astrocytosis is a specific feature.

ALMEIDA: Can I answer a question which Dr Dick asked, what I mean by transformed? I think Shine showed with SB40 in 1965 that if you put SB40 into human astrocytes which are growing in tissue culture, they suddenly begin to grow much more profusely. This isn't necessarily a malignant change in the sense that it is infiltrative, but it is a change which promotes rapid division of cells which may be very damaging to the patient, particularly when it occurs in the brain.

BECK: I have no cases of early Kuru. I had a few early Scrapies. But I can go one better in answering Dr Webb's question, and I am very glad he asked it. I speak only of natural Scrapie because Pattison has given a very beautiful demonstration of the sequence of events after the inoculation of Scrapie material. I was interested in what happens first so I asked Dr Parry a number of years ago for various sheeps' brains. Figs. 30–35, pp. 142–3, show sections all taken from exactly the same region of the upper brain stem. Figure 30 shows the normal astrocyte picture, from a clinically normal four and three quarter year old (non susceptible) sheep. Figure 31 was from an ancient, non-susceptible sheep (eight and a half years old), too old for breeding but clinically normal. There are proliferating astrocytes and from this figure one might well be led to diagnose Scrapie. Figure 32 is from a two and three quarter year old non-susceptible sheep which had anaemia and *post partum* pituitary necrosis. Here again astrocytic hypertrophy and proliferation is clearly shown.

Thanks to Dr Parry's genetic studies we now have twins of Scrapie parents one of whom was left to develop the disease and the other killed shortly before the disease in the twin showed itself. We might call the latter a 'pre-clinical' animal. Figure 33 is from such a pre-clinical sheep. It shows no astrocytic reaction. Figure 34 is from a normal animal of nonsusceptible stock which had a nodule in the lungs. This slide also shows clear astrocytic change which might lead to a diagnosis of Scrapie. Finally Fig. 35 is from a known case of Scrapie, moribund at the time of death. It shows characteristic astrocytic proliferation and hypertrophy. I do not think anyone can see a clear difference between Figs. 35, 34, 32 and 36.

I also examined the cerebellum in some of the pre-clinical animals. Figure 36 shows what we found. There were degenerating mossy endings in the cerebellum and that was the only change; at that stage there was no astrocytic reaction at all. We know that many of the afferent fibres from nuclei of the brainstem to the cerebellum end with mossy endings on the granule cells of the cerebellar cortex. Although it is not possible to determine from histological evidence alone, whether the fault lies at the site of the synapse with the granule cell or in the cells of origin in the brainstem, none of which were vacuolated, I thought these observations would give a pointer to those working on this question and I am glad to have had the chance of mentioning them.

SPILLANE: Dr Parry mentioned that although the Scrapie sheep could scarcely stand or walk they remain sexually active. In view of the description of the green monkey virus in Hamburg and in Jugoslavia and its possible transmission in seminal fluid, what is the possibility of sexual transmission here?

PARRY: We have got a lot of evidence that it is not transmitted by coitus and there have been many attempts to demonstrate the presence of the transmissible agent in seminal fluid and in blood and in saliva which have all been negative.

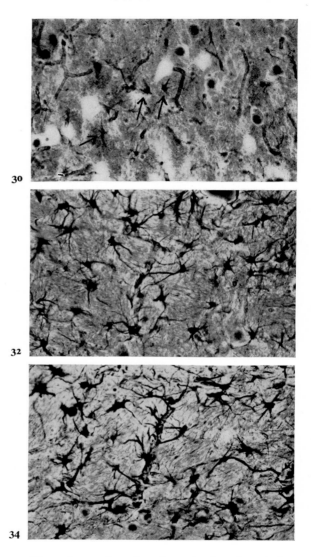

30

32

34

Figures 30–35. Photomicrographs taken from the lateral geniculate body of six sheep, only one of which was affected with Scrapie. Nos. 30, 31, 32 and 34 were from breeds not affected by Scrapie and from flocks where Scrapie has not occurred; all animals were neurologically normal. Nos. 33 and 35 were from breeds affected by Scrapie and from an affected flock. 30. F/4¾ years, clinically normal, killed as control; 31. F/8½ years, clinically normal, killed (too old for breeding); 32. F/2¾ years, anaemia associated with post-partum pituitary necrosis, killed; 33. F/3¼ years, clinically normal, potential Scrapie (progeny developed Scrapie), killed;

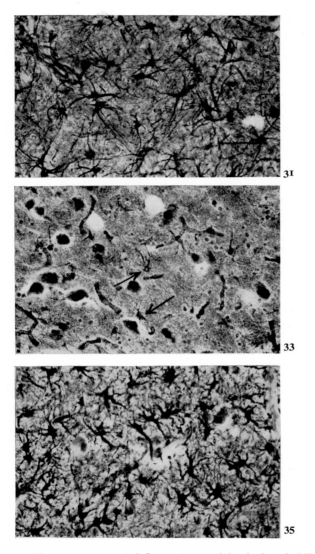

34. F/3 years, pregnant (inflammatory nodules in lungs), killed; 35. F/4 years, Scrapie, moribund, killed.
Note that astrocytic hypertrophy and proliferation is not confined to 35 (Scrapie), but is almost equally severe in 31, 32 and 34 (various clinical conditions non-Scrapie). By contrast 33 (pre-clinical Scrapie) shows only protoplasmic astrocytes (arrows), normal in number and appearance and not different from the normal control 30. In a further four cases of potential Scrapie astrocytes also appeared normal, in one their number was slightly increased. Cajal's gold-sublimate impregnation, × 200.

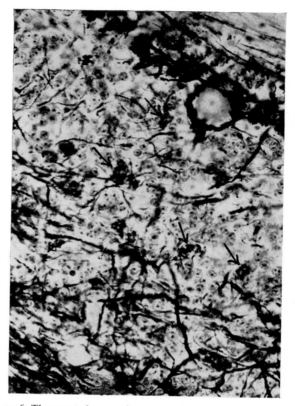

FIGURE 36. The same sheep as in Fig. 33. Cerebellum: The only pathological change found in this case was a widespread degeneration of mossy
endings (arrows) within the granular layer of the cerebellum. In a further
five cases of potential Scrapie degenerated mossy endings were also found.
Gros-Bielschowsky silver impregnation, × 480.

WATERSON: So far as the African green monkey virus goes there was
only one case in which they thought a man had transmitted it to his
wife. Virus was found in his semen, but this does not prove that
method of transmission: because they were in continuous domestic
contact in various ways all the time. We should not base too much on
one case.

ALMEIDA: Dr Alpers, has the known break in cannibalism given you a
chance to determine a time lag? You say that the disease was starting

at the age of four and is now at the age of 11. Have you definite information about this time lag and how does it affect the sex incidence? If we presume that the younger children are all infected, why, if there is a time lag which at the moment would seem to be as much as seven years, should you get a sharp break off of incidence in the male population?

ALPERS: The adult males have never been susceptible to the disease as far as we know and we postulated the differential cannibalism to explain this. The children of both sexes would have cannibalized with their mothers and this would explain the equal sex incidence amongst children. As the young boys left their mothers and went with their fathers at about the age of six, this took them out of the risk of infection. Since cannibalism has declined, we would expect that finally the whole disease would disappear. It should certainly disappear amongst children born since cannibalism stopped. We could say that the adults almost certainly cannibalized up to 1957 and as cases are still present we could postulate a long incubation period. This does not affect the sex ratio. That is explained by the fact that the males did not cannibalize beyond the age of six. If we want to look further into incubation periods on this hypothesis, it would seem that the minimum incubation period would be about three to five years because a cohort could either be infected *in utero* as the mother cannibalized, or else as they grew up and started eating solid food. So the ages of 0 and about two would be critical. We would expect that cohort to start coming down with the disease after the end of the minimum incubation period. Since the disease began about the age of four or five, the minimum incubation period on that analysis would be between three and five years. However we know the incubation period could have been longer, in fact probably was, because the equal sex ratio persisted until about the age of 18. Now the males left their mothers about the age of six, so this would mean a 12 year incubation period. At the moment this fits with the fact that age of onset in the younger age group is creeping up, till it is now about 12 years after the cannibalism ceased.

EARL: I would like to ask how Dr Parry was able to find out the genotype of the sheep; presumably from their past breeding record, and association or lack of association with any Scrapie in their lives?

PARRY: It is dangerous to make assumptions about genotypes on previous performances. You can use this as an hypothesis to see whether the data looks as if it is going to fit, then you must confirm in the following way. You have animals of the ss genotype which, mated with anything else, must produce heterozygous (*Ss*) off-spring, which we call 'greys' for brevity. We also have a small number of individuals with two affected parents, i.e. of genotype *ss* which we call 'blacks'. Then an unknown ram is taken and mated with 'black' ewes so as to give us enough progeny to allow six to be kept to four and a half years of age. If none of the six are affected this will give us a probability that the unknown ram is of *SS* genotype of about 1 in 100. If you mate with grey ewes you want about 22 progeny kept to the age of four and a half years for this probability. By various proportions you finish up with between six and 20 progeny and this is the basis for determining the primary genotypes. We call a proven homozygons dominant ram 'white'.

LEGG: Dr Alpers, have you a detailed cannibalistic history for the Foré inhabitants now, which might have some prediction value? Obviously not everyone has an equal chance of eating infected relatives, grandparents or parents, the number of relatives you eat depends on their life span and whether you are a boy and leaving home at six and so on. Are these facts known so that you could make some prediction for instance as to how many relatives you need to have eaten?

ALPERS: This may be difficult because if you go to the Foré now and ask about cannibalism, they will say 'cannibalism, never heard of it'! This all has to be done by digging up the past through informants who are willing to talk and we can get no precise data. We know there has been no cannibalism since 1957, or if there has been it's been in isolated areas. The younger cases are found now only in those isolated areas. For a while since 1957 incidence of Kuru in these areas was on the increase, now it seems generally to be on a slow decline.

PARRY: May I ask Dr Hunter or Dr Haig if they would comment on the fact that the transmissible agent from Scrapie seems to be widespread in many organs and yet it only seems to cause damage in the central nervous system? Or is this in fact not a true statement?

HAIG: No known histological changes have been demonstrated in any organ other than the central nervous system, but it is known that the transmissible agent is present to high titre, not quite so high as in the central nervous system, in spleen, lymph nodes and various glands. Perhaps there is a trace in blood but one is up against the technical difficulty of knowing whether or not a blood sample is contaminated. May I also raise a point about transformation of cells? Field's and some work by Pattison and myself has shown that astrocytes, or presumed astrocytes, in the affected brain of Scrapie mice can be grown more readily in tissue or organ cultures than material from normal mice. We have also found that it is comparatively easy to produce a cell line of brain cells, possibly glial, from Scrapie affected mice while it is extremely difficult to get this type of cell to grow from other mice. One can also demonstrate a clear difference between affected and normal brain by tryptonizing these preparations and on the following day noting a distinct difference in that the adherence of cells to the glass is far greater in the cultures from the Scrapie brain compared with the normal. The cells are different but I would hesitate to use the word transformed.

HUNTER: We have made some enzyme studies in other tissues and we haven't found any changes comparable to those we observed in brain. If I might supplement Mrs Beck's answer to an earlier question as far as the experimental disease is concerned, by far the earliest abnormality observed in Scrapie is the stimulation of DNA synthesis. This probably starts immediately after inoculation and reaches a maximum after four or five weeks. The change is confined to a small proportion, probably only about 0·1 % of the glial cells, but judging from measurements of nuclear size, both astrocytes and astroglia are affected.

ALPERS: I think the point Dr Parry has raised is important. It fits with my CIA (conditionally infectious agent). The importance of the metabolic requirements and genetic environmental background in the cell is critical here as to whether the agent is going to produce a disease or not. It looks as if Scrapie can be thought of as not only a slow virus in a very general way but also a latent one, depending on which cell it happens to be in. This brings up another point about the apparent non-immunogenicity of these agents. It is quite clear that Scrapie is proliferating in lymphnode cells from a very early stage so that if we are going to look for an antibody response we have to look very quickly, because the proliferation in this agent will lead to immunological paralysis. This will take place no matter what system we are using to protect antibody.

WEBB: Dr Hunter, could I just come back on this DNA synthesis. Didn't Stoker show that with polyoma virus the first thing that may occur is an increased DNA synthesis, before cell change or increased cell multiplication occurs? I am not sure whether you were supporting the idea that there might be some change in the cells or whether you were arguing against it. A second point, was there not some work at Compton in which the supernatant from Scrapie tissue cultures when put on normal brain cells produced more rapid growth?

HAIG: At Compton we have not had any success with this procedure. I think the work you referred to was done in the USA. Also in that same report an increased incidence of multinuclear cells was noted in cultures treated in that way. We have not confirmed this.

HUNTER: I would like to add that this increased DNA that we are measuring is not a part of the Scrapie agent, because it is confined to the nucleus of the cell and the Scrapie agent is extremely extra-nuclear.

CHAIRMAN: I think we must close this discussion. The lessons of Kuru and Scrapie seem to be growing and I was very interested to hear Dr Parry speak of a gene determined abiotrophy—a word that we thought had gone out a long time ago. Scrapie has an extraordinary resemblance to olivopontocerebellar degeneration and the whole question of systemic atrophies is broached. The astrocytic reaction in Kuru is not unlike what we see in multiple sclerosis: and Charcot was always interested in the primary role of the astrocyte in multiple sclerosis. In Kuru and Scrapie we have good reason to believe now that there is a replicating agent and it would be interesting to know how definitely it is affecting the astrocytes. Finally may I comment on the important case that Dr Matthews mentioned. It shows the value of team work; this work was carried out mostly in the USA but the biopsy was followed up in this country. I think it is an important case. There are I believe others in process of animal inoculation and we are waiting the results with great interest. Now I will ask Professor Dick to talk on subacute sclerosing panencephalitis.

Sub-Acute Sclerosing Panencephalitis

George Dick

Subacute sclerosing panencephalitis is a rare disease and during a ten year period (1956–1965) when I was in Northern Ireland there were three fatal cases recorded in the Department of Pathology of the University from a probable population of about 1·5 million. All of these occurred within a six months period in 1965. In the ten years prior to 1956, four fatal cases were recorded, three of which again occurred in a single year—1951 (Connolly 1968a). This gives some indication of the frequency and the grouping of these cases. Variously described as subacute sclerosing panencephalitis (SSPE), subacute sclerosing leukoencephalitis or inclusion body encephalitis, there is now a considerable amount of evidence that this condition is associated with infection of the CNS with a pseudomyxovirus, similar to or identical with measles virus. This is based on the original electron microscopic observations of Bouteille et al. (1965), and the antibody studies of Connolly et al. (1967), whose observations have been confirmed and expanded in several laboratories (see Zeman & Kolar 1968). Thus the electron microscope studies of Tellez-Nagel & Harter (1966), Herndon & Rubenstein (1968) and others have shown particles indistinguishable from paramyxoviruses budding from multitubular cytoplasmic inclusions, and secondly examination of brain sections with fluorescent antibody has shown particles of antigen, staining specifically with fluorescein labelled measles antibody which were distributed in cells in a manner that correlated with the inclusion bodies* (Lennette et al. 1968). There is little evidence to support the hypothesis that other viruses are involved in SSPE and the failure to find inclusion bodies in the brains of some patients does not exclude the possibility that measles or a closely related virus is the cause of this disease.

* Measles and distemper viruses are immunologically related as evidenced by the finding of distemper antibody in individuals who have been exposed to measles. Distemper virus is the only agent closely related to measles virus which is known to occur in the United Kingdom but no fluorescent staining of brains with conjugated distemper antibody has been demonstrated.

In addition to the electron microscope and fluorescent antibody studies additional evidence which implicates measles virus comes from antibody studies of cerebrospinal fluid and serum. The final proof by virus isolation has, however, not yet been obtained.

When I accepted Dr McCallum's invitation to talk at this meeting I told him that I had nothing to present, so what I shall be discussing is data from the workers in Northern Ireland and others. I would like in the first place to consider some observations on the levels of measles antibody in the serum and in the cerebrospinal fluid of patients with this condition and to discuss whether similar types of observations have helped or might help to clarify the aetiology of multiple sclerosis. Secondly, I shall review some attempts which have been made to isolate virus from the brains of patients with SSPE and, finally, mention the relevance of immunization against measles and this condition.

The levels of serum antibody to measles virus in patients with SSPE as measured by various techniques (Connolly *et al.* 1967, Connolly *et al.* 1968b, Lennette *et al.* 1968, Adels *et al.* 1968) have usually been considerably higher than is regularly seen after primary measles infection and in some cases where several samples have been tested throughout the illness, increases in the level of antibody have been found*. These observations suggest a continuous or repeated antigenic stimulus over a period of time.

In addition to these high levels of serum antibody, high levels of antibody to measles virus have been found in the cerebrospinal fluids. There are several possible explanations for this. In the first place, there may be an increased transfer of γ-globulin from serum to CSF as a result of an increased permeability of the blood brain barrier. Thus, Sherwin *et al.* (1963) and others have shown that inflammatory states of the CNS may result in an increased permeability of the blood/CSF barrier. If an increased permeability were the explanation of the high levels of measles antibody in the CSF then one might expect an increased permeability to other viral antibodies, unless there was a selective filtration of measles antibody. The serum CSF antibody ratios to measles virus in 18 patients with SSPE for whom data is available is calculated to be 16 : 1, e.g. the serum titre might be 1 : 2048 and that of the CSF 1 : 128. This is to be compared with a serum : CSF antibody

---

* In one patient who recovered Dr Legg (1967) reported that there was a drop in CF antibody although the HI titre persisted. It could be of value to measure the antibody levels in these patients at intervals; a drop in antibody might suggest a more hopeful prognosis than usual.

ratio of about 500 : 1 in normal individuals as measured with poliovirus antibodies (Clarke *et al.* 1965).

A comparison of the titres of type 2 poliovirus (neutralizing) antibody and of measles (haemagglutinin-inhibiting) antibody in the serum and CSF of three patients studied by Connolly, (1968b) is given in Table 13.

TABLE 13. Comparison of antibody titres* to type 2 poliovirus and to measles virus in three patients with SSPE (Connolly 1968b)

Patient		I	2	3
Polio	serum	362	1448	362
antibody	c.s.f.	< 2	< 2	< 2
	ratio	> 181	> 724	> 181
Measles	serum	2048	1024	64
antibody	c.s.f.	128	64	16
	ratio	16	16	4

* Figures are the reciprocals of dilutions.

The most likely explanation of these findings is that the excess of CSF measles antibody in patients with SSPE results from synthesis of immunoglobulins in the CNS.

It might be suggested that there is a selective permeability to measles antibody in patients with SSPE, however, increased selective transfer of measles antibody from the serum to CSF seems unlikely from the studies of Cutler *et al.* (1968) who have shown that when patients with SSPE were injected with radioactive IgG prepared from human serum or from CSF the patterns of the transfer from serum and CSF through the blood brain barrier were similar as far as the time and extent of equilibration, etc., were concerned.

A third possible explanation mentioned by Cutler *et al.* (1968) is that there has been fragmentation of γ-globulin in the CNS but from ultracentrifugal analysis they found no evidence of this.

It is of interest to enquire in passing whether there is evidence that antibody to measles virus may also be synthesized by cells in the CNS of patients with multiple sclerosis. Measles virus first came into the picture several years ago when it was shown that in groups of patients with multiple sclerosis the mean serum titres of measles virus antibody are higher than in control patients (Adams & Imagwa (1962), Reed *et al.* (1964), Sibley & Foley (1963), Clarke *et al.* (1965); Pette & Kuwert (1965)). It will be recalled that Kabat *et al.* (1942) showed that in most patients with multiple sclerosis the per cent of globulin in the CSF is raised while that of the serum was normal, and recently Tourtellotte *et al.* (1968) have shown that in the brain of a multiple sclerosis patient there is a greater amount of immunoglobulin-G than in normal brains while the concentration of albumin is similar. Tourtellotte *et al.* suggested that IgG is synthesized in the CNS of patients with multiple sclerosis and that this is reflected by an increase of IgG in the CSF.* Is there any evidence of an increase of measles virus antibody in the elevated brain γ-globulin? If it were shown that in multiple sclerosis patients the serum : CSF measles antibody ratios were much lower than the serum : CSF polio antibody ratios, then one might consider that there was local production of measles antibody in the CNS of multiple sclerosis as in SSPE. In order to get a base line Clarke *et al.* (1965) studied the poliovirus CSF : serum antibody ratios in groups of multiple sclerosis patients and in matched controls. They showed that in multiple sclerosis patients, the serum : CSF antibody ratios to polioviruses had a geometric mean titre of about half that of the control patients. Since there is no suggestion that polioviruses have anything to do with the aetiology of multiple sclerosis these lower than normal ratios are presumably due to damage to the blood brain barrier.

Due to technical problems, the measles serum : CSF ratios were not determined by Clarke *et al.* (1965), and data on this point from other laboratories is conflicting. It suggests either that the blood barrier is not equally permeable to the antibodies to polio, and to measles viruses, which I have already said is unlikely, or that the CSF contains a substance other than specific antibody capable of neutralizing measles virus. This problem requires further investigation.

While it is well known that it is difficult to isolate viruses from CNS after the acute stage of an infection it is perhaps surprising that virus has not been recovered from patients with SSPE, with the exception of one isolation in monkeys by Pelc *et al.* (1958). There may be two main reasons for these failures. In the first place, it may be that any infectious virus present is immediately neutralized by antibody and/or by other virus inhibitory substances in the CNS. Perhaps someone will be able to suggest how this problem can be overcome. One method is to trypsinize the infected material and then to seed tissue cultures with viable

---

* In confirmation, Cohen & Bannister (1967) have shown that lymphatic cells from CSF can synthesize IgA and IgG.

infected CNS cells rather than to homogenize the cells first, which could result in any virus which is liberated becoming inactivated by antibody. Secondly, by using living infected cells, the infective agent could spread to tissue culture cells by contact even if no infective virus were released. Alternatively, attempts might be made to isolate virus from long maintained tissue explants, and the starting material might first be treated with inactive measles vaccine virus to mop up any antibody or other neutralizing substances present. I am sure some of the virologists present will be able to suggest other techniques. The second reason is that it is of course possible that the measles virus infection of the CNS in patients with SPPE is a defective or abortive one, of which there are numerous examples in tissue culture systems. In some persistent defective infections of tissue cultures there may be little or no release of demonstrable virus or if it is released it may have lost virulence or infectivity. Rustigan (1966) has described persistent measles virus infections of HeLa cells grown in the presence of antibody where there was a continuous synthesis of intra-cellular viral antigen and intracytoplasmic inclusion bodies but no recoverable infectious virus. One such infected culture has been maintained for over six years with many hundreds of cell generations. If SSPE represents an aberrant type of adaptation of measles or of a measles-like myxovirus to neural tissue, it is difficult to see how the normal cycle can be restored.

A second type of approach might be to use some of the CNS material as antigen which could be injected into animals with or without adjuvants in order to immunize them or to boost an established immunity. It might be possible in this way to find out which antigens of measles virus, biopsy or autopsy material contained. Other techniques such as inhibition of the migration of measles-sensitive guinea-pig peritoneal cells by CNS tissue or blast cell transformation of measles-sensitive lymphocytes with CNS tissue have also been proposed (Paterson 1968).

Finally, will the widespread introduction of attenuated measles vaccine have any influence on the incidence of SSPE? There is one report of a child developing SSPE three weeks after receiving live measles vaccine (Schneck 1968) but in the present context, one is not concerned with acute complications but with the possibility of SSPE developing years after immunization. As a result of widespread measles vaccination and the subsequent reduction of 'wild' measles virus in the community it is to be hoped that SSPE will become even more uncommon and finally disappear from immunized communities. In order to find out if this is going to happen, careful surveillance will be required over the next 10 to 20 years. There are two important points to consider. As far as I know, one requirement of all experimental studies of defective infections, has been that the starting material has been grown in cells of a species different from the one used to maintain the persistent infection, although it has not been demonstrated that this is necessary (Fraser 1967): the original cells being competent and the recipient ones incompetent to allow maturation of virus. Is it probable that laboratory grown measles virus will more readily become defective than 'wild' virus when transmitted to man? Secondly, is there any evidence that attenuated measles viruses, similar in properties to vaccine viruses, are more frequently associated with SSPE than more virulent viruses? I think a number of people have been struck by the fact that cases of SSPE tend to occur in clusters although the patients have had no known contact. The three patients whom I saw in Northern Ireland in 1965 became ill within six months of each other and each of them had clinical measles between October 1952 and July 1953. In Northern Ireland epidemics of measles have occurred regularly every two years, the epidemic which was expected in 1952/3 did not take place (Connolly 1968).

In conclusion, may I say that while personally I believe that measles vaccine should have been introduced for selective immunization, now that it is being made available for general use, it is essential, although we cannot forecast the future, to ensure the maximum coverage possible, otherwise we shall build up a group of susceptible adolescents and adults who have escaped both immunization and natural infections. Such a population would, I think, be at greater risk of a severe illness if exposed to a virulent wild virus than to any potential risk associated with attenuated measles vaccine viruses.

REFERENCES

ADAMS J.M. & IMAGAWA D.T. (1962) Measles antibodies in multiple sclerosis. *Proc. Soc. exp. Biol.*, 111, 562–566.
ADELS B.R., GAJDUSEK D.C., GIBBS C.J., ALBRECHT P. & ROGERS, NANCY (1968) Attempts to transmit subacute sclerosing panencephalitis and isolate a measles related agent, with a study of the immune response in patients and experimental animals. *Neurology*, 18, 1 (Part 2), 30–51.
BOUTEILLE M., FONTAINE C., VEDRENNE CL. & DELARUE J.Z. (1965) Sur un cas d'encephalite subaigue a inclusions. Etude anatomo-clinique et ultrastructurale. *Rev. neurol.* 118, 454–458.
COHEN S. & BANNISTER R. (1967) Immunoglobulin synthesis within the central nervous system in disseminated sclerosis. *Lancet*, i, 366–367.

CONNOLLY J.H. (1968a) in Conference on Measles virus and subacute sclerosing panencephalitis. Measles virus as etiological agent in SSPE. *Neurology*, **18**, 1 (Part 2), 28.

CONNOLLY J.H. (1968b) Additional data on measles virus antibody and antigen in subacute sclerosing panencephalitis. *Neurology*, **18**, 1 (Part 2), 87–90.

CONNOLLY J.H., ALLEN I.V., HURWITZ L.J. & MILLAR J.H.D. (1967) Measles virus antibody and antigen in subacute sclerosing panencephalitis. *Lancet*, **1**, 542–544.

CUTLER R.W.P., MERLER E. & HAMMERSTAD J.P. (1968) Production of antibody by the central nervous system in subacute sclerosing panencephalitis. *Neurology*, **18**, 1 (Part 2), 129–132.

FRASER K.B. (1967) Defective and delayed myxovirus infections. *Brit. Med. Bull.* **23** (2), 178–184.

HERNDON R.M. and RUBINSTEIN L.J. (1968) Light and electron microscopy observations on the development of viral particles in the inclusions of Dawson's encephalitis (subacute sclerosing panencephalitis). *Neurology*, **18**, 1 (Part 2), 8–20.

KABAT E.A., MOORE D.H. & LANDOW H. (1942) Electrophoretic study of protein components in cerebrospinal fluid and their relationship to serum proteins. *J. Clin. Invest.* **21**, 571–577.

LEGG N.J. (1967) Virus antibodies in subacute sclerosing panencephalitis: a study of 22 patients. *Brit. med. J.* iii, 350–352.

PATERSON P.Y. (1968) Measles virus antigen in human nervous tissue. *Neurology*, **18**, 1 (Part 2), 104–106.

PETTE, EDITH & KUWERT E. (1965) Evaluation of multiple sclerosis sera against measles antigen in the complement fixation test. *Arch. ges. Virusforsch.* **16**, 141–147.

REED D., SEVER J., KURTZKE J. & KURLAND L. (1964) Measles antibody in patients with multiple sclerosis. *Arch. Neurol. (Chicago)*, **10**, 402–410.

RUSTIGAN R. (1966) Persistent infection of cells in culture by measles virus. I. Development and characteristics of Hela sublines persistently infected with complete virus. *J. Bact.* **92**, 1792–1804.

SCHNECK S.A. (1968) Vaccination with measles and central nervous system disease. *Neurology*, **18**, 1 (Part 2), 79–82.

SHERWIN A.L., RICHTER M., COSGROVE J.B.R. & ROSE B. (1963) Studies of blood cerebrospinal fluid barrier to antibodies and other proteins. *Neurol. (Minneap)*, **13**, 113–119.

SIBLEY W.A. & FOLEY J.M. (1963) Measles antibodies in multiple sclerosis. *Trans. Amer. neurol. Ass.* **88**, 277–281.

TELLEZ-NAGEL I. & HARTER D.H. (1966) Subacute sclerosing leukoencephalitis: ultrastructure of intranuclear and intracytoplasmic inclusions. *Science*, **154**, 899–901.

TOURTELLOTTE W.W., PARKER J.A., HERNDON R.M. & CUADROS C.V. (1968) Subacute sclerosing panencephalitis: brain immunoglobulin-G, measles antibody and albumin. *Neurology*, **18**, 1 (Part 2), 117–121.

ZEMAN W. & KOLAR O. (1968) Reflections on the etiology and pathogenesis of subacute sclerosing panencephalitis. *Neurology*, **18**, 1 (Part 2), 1-7.

Pathological Findings in Subacute Sclerosing Panencephalitis

Ingrid Allen

This presentation cannot pretend to be a comprehensive account of the histopathological findings in subacute sclerosing panencephalitis—it is merely a description of the findings in three recent cases in Belfast which I hope may serve as a basis for further discussion.

All three patients were males under the age of 20 who presented with their neurological symptoms during 1965. The clinical findings and EEG changes in each case led to a firm diagnosis during life. The main interest was virological in that all three had measles-virus antibody in serum and cerebrospinal fluid. The virological findings have already been described (Connolly, Allen, Hurwitz & Millar 1967, 1968, Connolly 1968).

Histologically the accepted pathological changes were present. Meningeal reaction was slight but there was widespread diffuse perivascular inflammation involving the deeper layers of the cerebral cortex, the white matter, the basal ganglia, the midbrain, brainstem, and the cerebellar white matter. In one case the inflammation was asymmetrical in that the left cerebral hemisphere was much more severely involved and this finding accounted for corresponding asymmetry in the clinical signs. The inflammatory infiltrate (Fig. 37) consisted predominantly of plasma cells and lymphocytes.

The superficial cortical laminae were well preserved but in the deeper layers of the cortex numerous collections of astrocytes and microglial cells were present and groups of these can be seen in Fig. 38. Foci of neuronophagia were common and shrunken neurones could be identified in the cerebral cortex and in the brainstem. Alzheimer's neurofibrillary change although sometimes a feature of subacute sclerosing panencephalitis was not found.

In all three patients there was diffuse isomorphic gliosis of the white matter (Fig. 39) and this change was associated in two of the patients with general pallor of myelin staining and scanty liberation of neutral fat. In the third patient, destruction of myelin was massive and had produced argyrophilic myelin masses and large quantities of neutral fat in the white matter. Figures 40 and 41 are from this patient and show the beading of myelin sheaths and the presence of neutral fat within lipid phagocytes.

In addition in this case numerous protoplasmic astrocytes were present and a few of these as shown in Fig. 42 were binucleate. Oligodendrocytes in this case were difficult to demonstrate and there seemed to be a reduction in the number of these cells which were seen in isolation in the white matter rather than in chains. In this patient the degree of myelin damage was marked and was disproportionately greater than the neuronal loss and axis cylinder damage.

In two of the cases the lateral columns of the spinal cord showed pallor of myelin staining but this change was not associated with inflammation or severe gliosis and was thought to be secondary to cerebral degeneration.

Both neuronal and glial inclusions were present in all three cases. The neuronal inclusions were predominantly nuclear though cytoplasmic inclusions were also seen. In addition extracellular eosinophilic rounded hyaline bodies were present and it was thought that these might represent extruded inclusions. The smallest form of nuclear inclusion consisted of an intensely eosinophilic body of approximately the same size as the nucleolus but distinguishable from it. Classical Cowdry type A inclusions were relatively common and were surrounded by a clear halo without any radial spike formation (Fig. 43). Cytoplasmic inclusions were eosinophilic, sometimes multiple, though often solitary large hyaline masses compressing the nucleus.

Glial inclusions were usually nuclear though in a few cells cytoplasmic inclusions were also present. These inclusions were eosinophilic and were seen in astrocytes and in oligodendrocytes where they frequently filled the whole cell (Fig. 44).

The staining reactions of various types of inclusions varied slightly but all were eosinophilic though phloxinophilia was variable. The very small nuclear inclusions were intensely eosinophilic—the Cowdry Type A cytoplasmic inclusions were slightly less so. In an attempt to assess the histochemistry, sections were stained for DNA using the Feulgen reaction and for RNA using the methyl green pyronin method of Unna and Pappenheim. In all sections the Feulgen reaction was negative. The majority of inclusions stained positively with pyronin and this suggested that they contained RNA, this hypothesis was strengthened by the fact that prior treatment of sections with ribonuclease destroyed the positive staining.

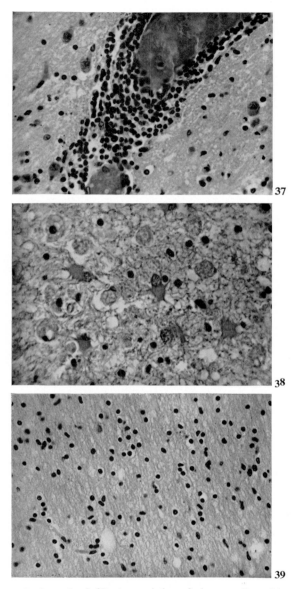

FIGURE 37. Perivascular infiltrate consisting of plasma cells and lymphocytes. Haematoxylin and eosin, × 400.

FIGURE 38. Protoplasmic astrocytes and lipid phagocytes in the deep white matter of the cerebral hemisphere. Haematoxylin and eosin, × 400.

FIGURE 39. Diffuse isomorphic gliosis of the white matter. Haematoxylin and eosin, × 300.

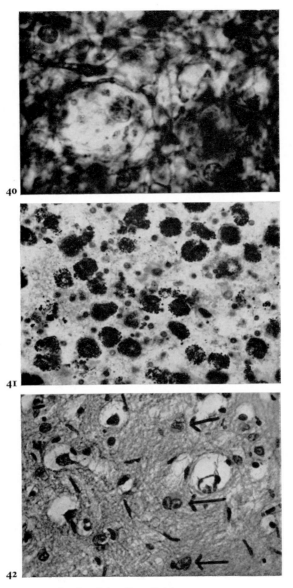

FIGURE 40. Myelin sheath beading. Spielmeyer, × 1300.
FIGURE 41. Neutral fat in lipid phagocytes. Scharlach R., × 400.
FIGURE 42. Binucleate astrocytes in the white matter. Haematoxylin and eosin, × 400.

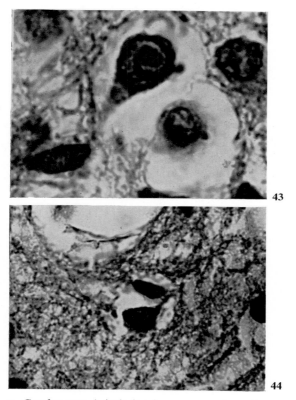

FIGURE 43. Cowdry type A inclusion in a neurone from the temporal cortex. Haematoxylin and eosin, × 1300.

FIGURE 44. Oligodendrocyte containing an intranuclear inclusion. Haematoxylin and eosin, × 1300.

In all three cases the presence of measles virus antigen within the brain was demonstrated using the direct fluorescent technique with patients' sera and goat antimeasles serum. The techniques used to establish specificity of fluorescent staining have already been described (Connolly *et al.* 1968).

In summary the histopathological findings in these three cases are those generally accepted as characteristic of subacute sclerosing panencephalitis. The severe degree of demyelination in one of the cases, though not a common finding judging from the literature, has never-

Ingrid Allen

theless been previously recognized and may have resulted from severe damage to oligodendrocytes. The staining reactions of the inclusion bodies suggest that they contain RNA and this finding is in keeping with the demonstration of measles virus antigen within brain cells.

REFERENCES

CONNOLLY J.H., ALLEN, INGRID V., HURWITZ L.J. & MILLAR J.H.D. (1967) Measles virus antibody and antigen in subacute sclerosing panencephalitis. *Lancet*, i, 542–544.

CONNOLLY J.H., ALLEN, INGRID V., HURWITZ L.J. & MILLAR J.H.D. (1968) Subacute sclerosing panencephalitis. *Quart. J. Med.* N. S. **37**, 625–644.

CONNOLLY J.H. (1968) Additional data on measles virus antibody and antigen in subacute sclerosing panencephalitis. *Neurology (Minneap.)* **18**, Part 2, 87–89.

Measles as an Aetiological Agent in Encephalitis

N.J.Legg

This is not a formal paper, but an introduction to discussion about the relationship between measles virus and the brain, as we see it clinically and as far as we understand it pathologically. As clinicians we are primarily concerned to disrupt the virus/host relationship in the host's favour, and in the laboratory viruses are maintained at the expense of other animal tissues, sometimes human. A more detached biological viewpoint, as in Dr Alpers' diagram (see Fig. 20, p. 93) is thus a necessary way of coordinating our information.

From the clinical point of view measles is an acute upper respiratory tract infection which is usually uncomplicated. We know, however, that if the CSF is examined it very frequently contains an increased number of inflammatory cells, and that if EEG tracings are taken before as well as after the appearance of the rash all patients show some abnormality. So this may well be a rash of the brain as well as of the skin: it may be a mild encephalitis or meningitis or possibly ependymitis. Measles can therefore certainly be classified on the diagram as an acute infection of the brain, with 'all or none' cell death.

Acute measles encephalitis may occur either early or late in the disease, and may sometimes precede the rash. It could be that the early cases are due to a proliferation of the virus in the central nervous system, and the later ones to an abnormal response of the brain to the antigen-antibody reaction which by then is undoubtedly being mounted. I don't think we have any evidence on that at the moment.

In subacute sclerosing encephalitis there is a very variable latent period between the original measles and the onset of the neurological illness; all the patients on whom we have information at the moment seem to have had ordinary acute measles at some time. Such a variable latent period occurs also with other latent virus infections such as varicella-zoster. As far as can be told there was nothing remarkable about the original attacks, nor was there a large incidence of encephalitis in the epidemics in which the patients suffered their attacks to suggest an unusually neurotropic strain.

The suggestion that such a neurotropic strain might account for acute measles encephalitis, as opposed to a mild ependymitis in ordinary measles, is lent some support by the work of Johnson & Johnson (1968) on another myxovirus. They inoculated suckling hamsters intracerebrally with mumps virus, using both unadapted and neuro-adapted strains. Seven days after inoculation the brains were stained with fluorescent antibody to show the distribution of virus antigen: with the unadapted strain this was confined to the ependymal cells, but with the neuro-adapted strain it was present in the neurones of the cerebral tissue.

Pathological evidence on the nature of measles encephalitis has been amplified in recent years by Adams (1968), who has found cytoplasmic and nuclear inclusion bodies in 75% of acute early measles encephalitis, and small multinucleate giant cells in about 25%, which he considers are indicative of measles virus invasion.

As far as the virology of subacute sclerosing encephalitis is concerned we know that it is associated with high measles antibodies in both the blood and the CSF. The former suggests that there is a viraemia at some stage, and the levels of the latter indicate that there is local production of antibodies in the brain as well. The two possible patho-geneses which we suppose for this are, firstly, a latent infection, follow-ing ordinary acute measles, which is reactivated in some fashion; and secondly a re-infection, perhaps with a measles virus which is more

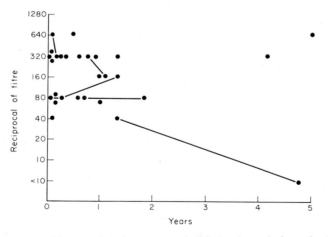

FIGURE 45. Subacute sclerosing panencephalitis. Reciprocal of measles CF antibody titre related to duration of neurological disease in years in 22 patients.

neuroadapted than the usual strain. Figure 45 shows the reciprocal of measles complement-fixing antibody in 22 patients, plotted against the duration of neurological symptoms. I didn't find any example in these patients comparable to the most instructive case which was studied in Belfast, with a progressively rising titre as the months went by, but in this figure is included an interesting boy of 18 who has now recovered and is in his 20's, whose complement-fixing antibody has fallen to an

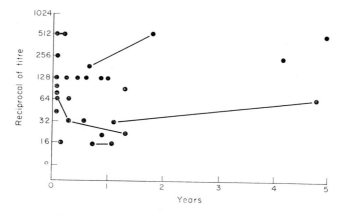

FIGURE 46. Subacute sclerosing panencephalitis. Reciprocal of measles HAI antibody titre related to duration of neurological disease in years in 22 patients.

undetectable level. Figure 46 shows similar data for haemagglutination-inhibiting antibodies, and this particular patient's titre has remained substantially unchanged: this is what one expects after a normal measles infection.

Returning to a consideration of the diagram (Fig. 20), we have to consider that measles can cause acute all-or-none cell death, either in the nasopharynx and respiratory tract alone or also in the brain; the possibility that it becomes latent and later is released to produce a slow infection which is progressive, causing degeneration of the brain's non-proliferating cell population; and the possibility of a reinfection with a slightly different form of measles virus, under the heading 'Temperate'. As a final speculation, we might fit multiple sclerosis into this picture by recalling the overgrowth of astrocytes which is an early feature of this condition, and suggesting that this could be regarded as a subdivision of the 'Neoplasia' section, resulting from

partially integrated RNA virus infection. It is clear that, as Dr Alpers
has already said, a virus can be fully discussed only in terms of its
relationship to its host.

REFERENCE

ADAMS J. (1968) Clinical pathology of measles encephalitis. *Neurology*, **18**, 2, 52.
JOHNSON R.T. & JOHNSON K.P. (1968) Myxoviruses and infections of the nervous
   system. *Neurology*, **18**, 2, 101.

Discussion on Subacute Sclerosing Panencephalitis

CHAIRMAN: McMENEMY: Dr van Bogaert, it's a privilege to have you here. You have a very long experience of this disease. Are there any comments you would like to make in relation to these recent views?

VAN BOGAERT: I have nothing to add to the actual problem: but I would like to say something about virus isolation. You will remember the early case of a girl from whom brain material was inoculated to a monkey. I have seen those slides and the picture in the monkey was not entirely similar to leucoencephalitis. Later on they tried to inoculate from this monkey's brain to another monkey. This second inoculation gave a picture like an acute poliomyelitis: as did the spinal cord. On enquiry it appeared later that the second monkey was living for two or three weeks in a room where there had been polio before: so it may be that his condition had nothing to do with that of the first monkey. I have also always been a bit reserved about the similarity of the first one's picture to leucoencephalitis.

DICK: One small point for the record, I didn't mean that people with subacute sclerosing encephalitis were reinfections. I believe that they are continuing infections. But the three patients whom I saw in 1965 in Northern Ireland became ill within six months of each other. Now in the year 1952/1953, the usual expected measles epidemic with brain involvement did not occur in the community. I was therefore postulating that perhaps a more virulent or less virulent virus was in the community during that year and was responsible for these cases of subacute sclerosing encephalitis.

VAN BOGAERT: May I add that in leucoencephalitis, whether dying after six months or after four or five years, you find just the same histological picture.

MATTHEWS: I think clinicians here would be interested to know for the future exactly what specimens or information virologists require in order to help with the diagnosis.

MacCallum: I think that one of Dr Alpers' pamphlets has actually got this information listed. May I ask Dr Dick a technical question? One patient of Dr Whitty's seemed to fit in to this group due to measles, but serum for the haemagglutination inhibiting tests sent to Dr Clarke of the Medical Research Council was negative. We therefore thought this was not measles associated. A few weeks ago she wrote to say that she had retested this serum without absorption on kaolin, and got positive results. Does this mean that this is a different specific antibody or not?

Dick: This is a very technical problem and I don't know yet. We need to do a lot more work on it. Whether or not she got two antibodies would depend on the level of the serum antibody to some extent.

Alpers: About specimens for the virologist; any interesting and unusual neurological condition should have some material put away frozen, taken as soon after death as possible; as well as serum and CSF, which should be cold stored and not thrown out. These can be useful even after long storage.

Webb: About antibodies and the CSF, we have been interested in this in humans with cancer who have been treated with virus. Gordon Smith found that by adding a little bovine albumin to the CSF protein, the haemagglutination test previously negative became as strongly positive as it was in the blood.

Urich: May I mention a strange case of SSPE that I saw. It was of a child who developed the disease at the age of about one year some two or three weeks after immunization with the standard triple vaccine.

The disease ran a typical clinical course and was diagnosed clinically, but during its course about a month or so before her death the child developed a typical clinical measles which then cleared up. At autopsy the brain histologically would have passed as multiple sclerosis. It showed an inflammatory reaction of the cortex, and a very severe degree of cerebellar atrophy, but no inclusion bodies. Where does a case like this fit in?

Chairman: If no one can give a rapid answer to this we must close this discussion. I will ask Dr Webb and then Dr Wells to talk.

The Pathogenesis of the Viral Encephalitides

H. E. Webb

As the purpose of this meeting is to put forward ideas and to promote discussion it seemed right to try and summarize one's own ideas on the mechanisms involved in the pathogenesis of the viral encephalitides. Because of time it is impossible to go into great detail of the experimental and theoretical background for the hypothesis put forward but it is hoped that where relevant these facts may be considered in any discussion.

Types of encephalitis
These may be divided into acute and chronic: the acute encephalitides occurring within one month of the infection; the chronic occurring at a time later than this, perhaps months or years. The acute encephalitides may progress to become chronic. In the first group would be included infections with poliomyelitis, arboviruses, adenoviruses, chicken pox, measles, herpes and many others. In the second group herpes is again involved and in the light of recent work probably measles also in what has come to be named subacute sclerosing panencephalitis (SSPE) (Bouteille *et al.* 1965, Connelly *et al.* 1967). The role of viruses in the chronic encephalitic states of post encephalitic parkinsonism and in progressive multifocal leucoencephalopathy (PMLE) (Howatson *et al.* 1965) has still to be determined. Also to be included in this group, if a viral aetiology is finally established, will be such diseases as kuru and multiple sclerosis.

Cells within the central nervous system (CNS) differ in their susceptibility to virus infections and the viruses themselves are selective also. For example, paralytic poliovirus infections show lesions particularly of motor neurone cells, the arboviruses the cells of the grey matter and herpes simplex of both grey and white matter. The pathology in these acute infections will differ but the mechanisms involved may be very similar. Viruses not only cause destructive lesions but they may also be involved in stimulating cells to excess growth. How this may play a part in the pathogenesis of the encephalitides is discussed later.

The passage of virus to the CNS

Experimentally viruses can spread to the CNS via the peripheral nerves either by multiplication in the endoneural or perineural cells or by more rapid diffusion without evidence of cellular infection, in a similar way from the olfactory mucosa or by direct invasion of the arachnoid cuffs surrounding the nerves within infected sub-mucosal tissue. However the most likely method and the one of the greatest importance in naturally occurring human encephalitis is by the distribution of virus particles by the blood to the CNS (Johnson & Mims 1968).

The importance of the viraemia

Almost certainly all viruses cause a general infection before the CNS is involved. Even in those virus infections which have been termed 'neurotropic' clinical involvement of the CNS is rare, though it must be stressed that the CNS is infected in virus diseases a great deal more often than is clinically apparent. Mumps is a good example of this (Meyer *et al.* 1960). The viruses which produce the biggest viraemia are likely to be those which most often cause acute encephalitis because:

1.   There is widespread distribution of a great many virus particles which increases the chances for those viruses which are able to multiply in CNS cells of finding these cells. It is of interest that Nathanson & Bodian (1962) stressed the importance of even minimal viraemia in the invasion of the CNS with polio virus. The Mahoney strain in monkeys, with its characteristically large viraemia regularly produced CNS invasion with very high paralytic rates.

2.   The large quantity of circulating virus particles will provoke, because of the quantity of antigen, a good antibody response which will make a clinically detectable disturbance of the CNS more likely.

The factors which cause the clinical syndromes

It is very important to stress that virus infection of a cell and virus multiplication within a cell is by no means synonymous with cell destruction. The tolerant infections with the lymphocytic-choriomeningitis virus is an excellent example of this phenomenon (Weigand and Hotchin 1961).

Two main processes seem to be involved in the CNS damage caused in the acute virus encephalitides.

1.   The second cycle of multiplication of virus in the cells of the CNS can destroy the particular type of cell infected. These cells vary depending on the selectivity of the virus involved.

2. The acute viral encephalitides do not show their CNS symptoms and signs until the viraemia is subsiding and antibody developing. The second factor, then, is the reaction of virus (antigen) with antibody producing inflammation and oedema. This probably starts in the walls of the small vessels increasing their permeability. The second virus multiplication cycle in the CNS begins soon after viraemia and this virus too will react with antibody leaking through the vessel walls. The possibility of these reactions being a hypersensitivity (allergic) type of reaction is discussed by Webb & Smith (1966). Webb *et al.* (1968a, 1968b) have put forward further evidence in support of these ideas. Hypersensitivity type reactions in virus diseases may not be associated with the CNS only as pointed out by Webb (1968).

How does this fit into the histological and clinical syndromes found?
If one believes that the blood stream spread of virus is the most important method of infecting the CNS, then one can postulate that during the second virus multiplication cycle there will be a build up of virus around the vessels followed by a 'zoning out' phase as the virus multiplies and spreads in the CNS. Virus multiplication then takes place in those cells especially suited for that particular type of virus. Also, at this time, with antibody leaking through these vessels from the blood, the two mechanisms of cellular destruction can take place and both will be directed at the site of maximal viral activity. With this hypothesis the intense perivascular infiltration with lymphocytes and plasma cells could be explained. It can also explain the grey matter involvement of many of the arbovirus infections and of the perivascular demyelination of the 'post-infective' encephalitides, e.g. measles and vaccinia, if these latter viruses have a higher rate of multiplication in the glial cell elements, the disturbance of which may cause a secondary demyelinization.

It is difficult to see oedema by histological or electron-microscopical means but this undoubtedly occurs in a hypersensitivity reaction because of the increased capillary permeability. Papilloedema is frequently seen in cases of severe encephalitis and this must result from cerebral oedema. The production of oedema in the CNS can cause secondary anoxia of cells by ischaemia. This, at first, may embarrass cellular function and then if allowed to continue produce death of cells. In those cases of poliomyelitis which have complete paralysis followed by complete recovery it seems likely that viral action has not been sufficient to destroy the cell but the combination of viral multiplication and its reaction with developing antibody causing oedema and anoxia had created a situation in which the function of the cell was disturbed but not beyond recovery. The factor of oedema could perhaps also explain why so often the most used limb in polio-myelitis becomes the most severely paralysed. Functioning anterior horn cells have a higher rate of metabolism than those at rest and therefore use more oxygen. If they are already embarrassed by intra-cellular virus multiplication and ischaemic from the pressure of sur-rounding oedema then the lack of extra oxygen when under stress from having to function, will result in cell death. So it seems that the inflammatory reaction and oedema from this hypersensitivity type reaction may play an important part in the pathogenesis of the acute encephalitides. Fell et al. (1966) and Dingle et al. (1967) have also shown that certain types of antigen-antibody reactions produce exces-sive metabolic activity though leaving the cell fully viable. The type involved is when complement and antibody react with cell membrane antigens. In this process the lysosomal system is activated and the enzymes released from the cells are damaging. Steroids have the ability to stabilize lysosomes and reduce the liberation of their acid hydrolases (Thomas 1964). Coombs (1968) goes further into the details of allergic reactions and their responsibility for disease and particularly refers to microbial pathogenesis in this respect. If this is the case then it is justifiable to try steroids in large doses for a short time at the onset of the encephalitic stage of the illness, because they are very good at reducing the oedema from a hypersensitivity type reaction. I use it and am personally convinced of its beneficial effect if used correctly. As steroids suppress the production of interferon (Kilbourne et al. 1961) and interferon is a defence mechanism against viruses it would be quite wrong to use them as a preventive for encephalitis. This would be tantamount to giving steroids during the viraemia when interferon is being produced. By giving them at the onset of the encephalitic phase both blood interferon and CNS interferon will have been pro-duced already thus these natural processes will not be affected.

Chronic viral encephalitis

It is becoming evident that many more viruses than previously thought have the capacity for latency. The arboviruses, particularly of the tick-borne complex, show this (Price 1966, Reeves et al. 1958, Reeves 1961). Herpes is well known for this particular property. If SSPE is confirmed as being due to measles virus then this will be another. Adenoviruses lie latent in tonsilar tissue (Israel 1962) and there are many other examples. So in chronic encephalitis one is facing a situation in which the CNS has become infected often silently to begin with and then at a later date symptoms and signs of a more chronic type of CNS disturbance develop. The possible mechanisms for this appear to be:

1.   There is a slow and steady destruction of cells by virus multiplication within them. This would seem the least likely as this would expose the virus to extracellular fluid antibodies which would neutralize it and prevent further infection. But in the CNS there may be a mechanism for passage of virus from cell to cell without going through extra-cellular fluid, e.g. measles virus can cause cell fusion both in tissue culture and *in vivo* (Enders *et al.* 1957, Warthin 1931). Fusion of CNS cells as a result of measles virus has not been described yet but a mechanism of this nature in both measles and other virus infections might explain how viruses can persist in the CNS.

2.   There is an upset in the status quo of the antigen (virus)-antibody relationship which may cause local inflammatory reactions with death of cells. Antibody has been measured in the cerebrospinal fluid (CSF) in many virus infections and Connolly (1968) has suggested a useful method of determining whether the antibody found there is likely to have been mostly produced in the CNS or resulted from a 'leak' through an inflamed or damaged 'blood-brain barrier'. It seems that both mechanisms for the presence of antibody in the CNS are accept-able. Incidentally, I am surprised that the clinicians, who want a definitive diagnosis, do not make more use of the fact that antibodies in the CSF rise later than in the blood. At the time a patient presents with the encephalitic phase of viral illness the blood antibodies are already high but the CSF antibodies are often negative. It may not be possible to show a further 4-fold rise in the blood haemagglutinating antibodies but it is very easy to do so using paired CSF samples parti-cularly if a little bovine albumen is added to increase the overall quan-tity of CSF protein.

It may be that during an intercurrent infection with an agent that produces meningeal inflammation blood antibody from a previous infection can leak through and react with the virus that is latent in the CNS. It is of interest in this respect that lesions are numerous in both the acute and chronic encephalitides around the vessels and ventricular systems. This is also the case in diseases such as multiple sclerosis. Is the reason for this because these are the areas where the maximum amount of antigen-antibody reactions are likely to take place?

3. A different type of antigen-antibody reaction may be taking place because of the ability of viruses to enter cells and incorporate themselves into the structure of that cell thus altering the cell's antigenicity and stimulating the host to reject the whole cell. This could well account for the slow destruction of cells in the CNS with raised globulins in the CSF and an auto-immune type of phenomenon.

4. The transformation of cells by viruses possibly causing excess gliosis and microgliosis is another possibility. That many viruses have the capacity to stimulate cells to multiply abnormally, i.e. 'transform' them, is certain and it is of great interest in relation to the CNS that Zlotnik (1968) has found particularly with arboviruses that one of the earliest changes in the brain is the hypertrophy and proliferation of the astrocyte. He has also shown that repeated viral stimulation intensifies this phenomenon. Miss S. J. Illavia in my department has shown that mouse brain tissue cultures will survive several months and the growing cells are not killed, nor do they have their growth rate decreased by the inoculation of large concentrations of at least two arboviruses (Langat and Kyasanur Forest disease). The cells, in fact, support the multiplication of these viruses for many weeks yielding considerable quantities of virus over this period. The amount of glial hypertrophy and proliferation seen in both chronic viral CNS disease and in those diseases suspected of having a viral aetiology such as Scrapie, Kuru and multiple sclerosis, is very impressive. This may well result from transformation of the glial elements by a virus or a part of a virus. The demyelination in these conditions I personally believe is secondary to the abnormalities of the oligodendrocyte and/or the astrocyte. Both these cells have been associated with the production of myelin. Peters (1964) has shown by electron microscopy the relationship of the oligodendrocyte and Wendell-Smith et al. (1966) the astrocyte to the development of myelin. Measles virus and others of the myxo virus group seem to have an affinity for glial cells and it is reasonable to suppose that the presence of virus particles in them might upset the conditions necessary for the myelin sheath which has been derived from them, to survive. There are many demyelinating diseases including 'multiple sclerosis' which probably have a viral aetiology. The aetiological agent in some cases of 'multiple sclerosis' may well be the measles virus, as suggested by the work of Adams & Imagawa (1962) and Pette (1968), if one can accept the glial cells as being an important site

of viral activity and therefore the centre of any abnormal process. This could be a primary destructive or proliferative process or secondarily destructive from the result of antigen-antibody reactions or each of these things concurrently. Each process individually may have the capacity to inhibit the cells' capacity to support the myelin it has produced. As many viruses or parts of virus may have the capacity to transform or destroy glial cells, the aetiological agents for the clinical syndromes of 'multiple sclerosis' are likely to be several though the mechanism of development of the lesions in each case may be similar.

Conclusion

I believe that, apart from the direct effect of viruses on cells a hypersensitivity type reaction plays a very important part in the pathogenesis of virus infections both with reference to the acute CNS syndromes seen and also in other virus diseases where the 'target' organ may be different. I believe this reaction may play a most important part in explaining the death of monkeys I inoculated with Kyasanur Forest disease (KFD) virus in some early experiments. Monkeys injected with KFD virus and which circulated this virus to a high titre frequently died towards the end of the viraemia on the eighth to fourteenth day at a time when antibodies were developing (Webb 1961). This is also the time when the pancytopaenia is recovering (Webb & Chatterjea 1962). Twenty-four to forty-eight hours before death the monkeys developed bradycardia, diarrhoea and hypotension. This is a clinical syndrome which suggests an acute autonomic nervous system disturbance similar to that seen on giving large doses of prostigmine intravenously and in states of anaphylactic shock. This was further investigated by Webb & Burston (1966) but histological examination of the CNS and autonomic nervous system revealed no abnormality by the ordinary techniques. No histochemical techniques were used. It is quite clear from the article by Coombs (1968) that antigen reacting with antibody particularly in his Type I and Type III reaction can liberate substances which produce anaphylaxis. The precise cause of death in these animals though still remaining a mystery I believe now to be caused by an acute antigen-antibody (hypersensitivity) type reaction with liberation of one of these substances.

As far as the chronic viral CNS syndromes are concerned I believe the most important factor to be the ability of many more viruses to become 'latent' than were previously thought. This, combined with the ability of a virus to do different things to cells under different circumstances and the body to respond to these changes with its own immunological reactions, produces chronic inflammatory reactions and cellular proliferation which is incompatible with the definitive function and survival of the normal CNS cells.

REFERENCES

ADAMS J.M. & IMAGAWA D.T. (1962) Measles antibodies in multiple sclerosis. *Proc. Soc. exp. Biol.* **111**, 562.

BOUTEILLE M., FONTAINE C., VEDRENNE C. & DELARUE J. (1965) Sur un cas d'encéphalite subaiguë à inclusions. Étude anatomoclinique et ultrastructurale. *Rev. neurol.* **113**, 454.

CONNOLLY J.H. (1968) Additional data on measles virus antibody and antigen in subacute sclerosing panencephalitis. *Neurology (Minneap.)* **18**, 87.

CONNOLLY J.H., ALLEN I.V., HURWITZ L.J. & MILLAR J.H.D. (1967) Measles virus antibody and antigen in subacute sclerosing panencephalitis. *Lancet,* i, 542.

COOMBS R.R.A. (1968) Immunopathology. *Brit. med. J.* i, 597.

DINGLE J.T., FELL B.B. & COOMBS R.R.A. (1967) The breakdown of embryonic cartilage and bone cultivated in the presence of complement-sufficient antiserum. 2. Biochemical changes and the role of the lysosomal system. *Int. Arch. Allergy*, **31**, 282.

ENDERS J.F., PEEBLES T.C., McCARTHY K., MILORANOVIC M., MITUS A. & HOLLOWAY A. (1957) Measles virus: a summary of experiments concerned with isolation, properties and behaviour. *Amer. J. Pub. Health*, **47**, 275.

FELL H.B., COOMBS R.R.A. & DINGLE J.T. (1966) The breakdown of embryonic (chick) cartilage and bone cultivated in the presence of complement-sufficient antiserum. 1. Morphological changes, their reversibility and inhibition. *Int. Arch. Allergy*, **30**, 146.

HOWATSON A.F., NAGAI M. & ZU RHEIN G.M. (1965) Polyoma-like virions in human demyelinating brain disease. *Canad. med. Ass. J.* **93**, 379.

ISRAEL M.S. (1962) The viral flora of enlarged tonsils and adenoids. *J. Path. Bact.* **84**, 169.

JOHNSON R.T. & MIMS C.A. (1968) Pathogenesis of viral infection of the nervous system. *New Engl. J. Med.* **278**, 23.

KILBOURNE E.D., SMART K.M. & POKORNY B.A. (1961) Inhibition by cortisone of synthesis and action of interferon. *Nature, Lond.* **190**, 650.

MEYER H.M. JR., JOHNSON R.T., CRAWFORD I.P., DASCOMB H.E. & ROGERS N.G. (1960) Central nervous system syndromes of 'viral' etiology. *Amer. J. Med.* **29**, 334.

NATHANSON N. & BODIAN D. (1962) Experimental poliomyelitis following intramuscular virus injection. III. The effect of passive antibody on paralysis and viraemia. *Bull. Johns Hopkins Hosp.* **111**, 198.

PETERS A. (1964) Observations on the connections between myelin sheaths and glial cells in the optic nerves of young rats. *J. Anat.* **98**, 125.

PETTE E. (1968) Measles virus: a causative agent in multiple sclerosis. *Neurology, (Minneap.)*, **18**, 168.

PRICE W.H. (1966) Chronic disease and virus persistence in mice inoculated with Kyasanur Forest disease virus. *Virology*, **29**, 679.

REEVES W.C. (1961) Overwintering of arthropod-borne viruses. *Progr. Med. Virol.* **3**, 59.

REEVES W.C., HUTSON G.A., BELLAMY R.R. & SCRIVANI R.P. (1958) Chronic latent infections of birds with western equine encephalomyelitis virus. *Proc. Soc. exp. Biol.* **97**, 733.

THOMAS L. (1964) In: *Injury, Inflammation and Immunity*, L.Thomas, J.W.Uhr & L.H.Grant (Eds.), Baltimore.

WEBB H.E. (1961) *Kyasanur Forest Disease in Animals and Man*, D.M. Thesis. Oxford.

WEBB H.E. (1968) Factors in the host virus relationship which may affect the course of an infection. Paper to Royal Society of Medicine meeting 2–3 May. *Brit. Med. J.* (in press).

WEBB H.E. & BURSTON J. (1966) Clinical and pathological observations with special reference to the nervous system in macaca radiata infected with Kyasanur Forest Disease virus. *Trans. roy. Soc. trop. Med. Hyg.* **60**, 325.

WEBB H.E. & CHATTERJEA J.B. (1962) Clinico-pathological observations on monkeys infected with Kyasanur Forest Disease virus, with special reference to the Haemopoietic system. *Brit. J. Haemat.* **8**, 401.

WEBB H.E. & SMITH C.E.G. (1966) Relation of immune response to development of central nervous system lesions in virus infections of man. *Brit. med. J.* ii, 1179.

WEBB H.E., WIGHT D.G.D., PLATT G.S. & SMITH C.E.G. (1968a) Langat virus encephalitis in mice. 1. The effect of the administration of specific antiserum. *J. Hyg., (Camb.)* **66**, 343.

WEBB H.E., WIGHT D.G.D., PLATT G.S., WIERNIK G. & SMITH C.E.G. (1968b) Langat virus encephalitis in mice. II. The effect of irradiation. *J. Hyg., (Camb.)* **66**, 355.

WEIGAND M. & HOTCHIN J. (1961) Studies of lymphocytic choriomeningitis in mice. II. A comparison of the immune status of newborn and adult mice surviving inoculation. *J. Immun.* **86**, 401.

WENDELL-SMITH C.P., BLUNT M.J. & BALDWIN F. (1966) The ultra structural characterisation of macroglial cell types. *J. comp. Neurol.* **127**, 219.

WARTHIN A.S. (1931) Occurrence of numerous large giant cells in tonsils and pharyngeal mucosa in prodromal stage of measles; report of 4 cases. *Arch. Path.* **11**, 864.

ZLOTNIK I. (1968) Reaction of astrocytes to acute virus infections of the central nervous system. *Brit. J. exp. Path.* (in press).

Types of Vaccinial Encephalopathy

C. E. C. Wells

During the mass prophylaxis of 1962, when smallpox was epidemic in South Wales, some 30 cases of central and nine cases of peripheral nervous disorder beginning near the peak of the vaccinial reaction were admitted to hospitals in the Cardiff area. Although the patterns of clinical disease were so varied, the prognosis was generally good and only one patient was known to have died (Spillane & Wells 1964).

Signs common to all cases were the vesicle of recent successful vaccination together with a zone of erythema, enlarged lymph nodes and fever. The distinction between cases of primary and secondary vaccination which is often made in accounts of post-vaccinial disorders was unimpressive as the two groups were evenly matched. A successful vaccination was taken as evidence of previous non-immunity which had enabled the virus to lodge at the inoculation site before its dissemination in a generalized vaccinia viraemia.

Encephalomyelitis

During the nineteen-twenties a specific neurohistological lesion was delineated in some cases dying in coma after Jennerian vaccination (Turnbull & McIntosh 1926, Bouman & Bok 1927, Perdrau 1928); and was later found in rare cases of other virus infections and of measles (de Vries 1960). The preceding neurological illness became known as post-vaccinial encephalomyelitis. Unfortunately Comby (1907) had used a similar title—'encéphalite aiguë vaccinale'—for an illness now believed to have a different pathogenesis; and subsequent reports of all neurological disorders after vaccination have used this diagnostic label.

The brain of the fatal case in the Cardiff series was found to have the typical changes of post-vaccinial encephalomyelitis: discrete areas of perivenous demyelination with proliferation of microglia throughout the central neuraxis, spinal cord, and white matter of the hemispheres, but with characteristic sparing of cortical neurones and absence of haemorrhage (de Vries 1960).

In ten of the Cardiff cases, including this patient (Case 7), the cardinal symptoms were clouding of consciousness and amnesia of several days' duration. Stupor, delirium, or coma, were ingravescent; other signs found in the majority were meningism, tremor, ataxia and involuntary movements such as chorea, ballism and oculogyric crises. During recovery from decorticate rigidity one patient (Case 8) developed transient bulimia and a high-pitched monotonous dysarthria, like that described in the encephalomyelitis of modified smallpox (Marsden & Hurst 1932).

Spinal symptoms were prominent in three cases and persisted long into convalescence (Cases 5, 6 and 10). Another patient (Case 11) had acute transverse myelitis which remitted rapidly and completely in the sixth week: despite the lack of cerebral symptoms or signs her disorder was thought to be typical of encephalomyelitis and she was included in this group.

Although the pressure of the spinal fluid was normal or only slightly raised, the contents were abnormal in eight of the 11 cases. The commonest finding was a lymphocytic pleocytosis (10 to 292 cells/cu mm) with a small rise of protein (usually below 100 mg, with maximum 140 mg/100 ml) and normal sugar. Cultures were consistently sterile and the Wassermann and related serological tests for syphilis negative.

Other laboratory tests were generally uninformative. Four cases had a moderate leucocytosis of the peripheral blood, and the vaccinia haemagglutination-inhibition test was positive in the five cases for whom it was requested.

Electroencephalograms recorded during the first fortnight were invariably abnormal with generalized high-voltage slow waves, of delta and sub-delta frequencies, appearing symmetrically in tracings from both hemispheres. A return to normal rhythms followed gradually in the wake of clinical recovery. Electroencephalograms were not taken in two cases; and were normal in four others from whom records could not be obtained during the acute phase of the illness.

Ten of the 11 cases diagnosed as encephalomyelitis survived. The oldest patient of the whole series, a 59-year-old widow, died of pulmonary embolism within 24 hours of her admission in coma with hyper-pyrexia. Seven patients recovered without sequelae. Spinal symptoms persisted in two others for some months and in a third signs of spastic paraparesis were still present shortly before she died two years later of unrelated mental disease.

Encephalopathy

Seven adults (Cases 15 to 21) were admitted to the local isolation hospital at the request of their general practitioners with a provisional diagnosis of encephalitis. Their illness, however, seemed to be essentially a benign accentuation of the usual symptoms of successful vaccination —headache, fever, photophobia, meningism. The spinal fluid contents were normal but in two cases the pressure was raised. Transient pulmonary shadows and conjunctivitis in three cases were thought to be due to the viraemia of vaccinia, to which the whole illness was attributed.

No infants with neurological symptoms were reported from Cardiff although certain types of skin disorder were frequent in this age group (Waddington, Bray, Evans & Richards 1964). Three children, however, aged six and a half, eight and a half and 11 years, became ill with symptoms and clinical signs which distinguished them from the cases of encephalomyelitis.

The illness of the two younger children (Cases 12 and 13) began abruptly with epileptic convulsions, followed in the elder by a transient hemiparesis, but with quick recovery of consciousness and return to normal within a few days. Amnesia was brief and limited to the period of post-epileptic confusion. Twelve days after vaccination the eldest child (Case 14) complained of colic and joint pains which were followed by urticaria, purpura, haematuria and bloody diarrhoea. Six days later she had a fit and was aphasic with right hemiplegia for the next week. She recovered fully.

In all three the pressure of the spinal fluid was normal, the contents being normal in two but the protein raised in the third. Electroencephalograms of the two patients with hemiparesis showed slow-wave foci of the opposite hemisphere and a diffuse disturbance in the youngest child who had had continuous one-sided twitching.

Three patients (Cases 22, 23 and 24) had a story only of epilepsy. A woman aged 34 had a single fit nine days after vaccination and a second episode of transient confusion, without known convulsion, a fortnight later. A nine-year-old girl was admitted to hospital with high fever after a nocturnal fit on the sixth day. Neither patient was given anticonvulsant therapy and both remained well without further incident. The third case, a girl of 13, was in petit mal status for five days. Drug therapy which seemed ineffective was withdrawn but she did not relapse.

Six patients (Cases 25 to 30) had an illness akin to demyelinating disease: three of them had had previous episodes and two were already attending hospital as cases of suspected multiple sclerosis.

Neuropathy

Five cases of polyneuritis (Cases 31 to 35) and two of brachial neuritis (Cases 36 and 37) were seen in addition to the 30 cases of central nervous disorder. In these seven cases the interval between vaccination and the onset of neurological symptoms (14 days) was a little longer than in the cases of encephalomyelitis and encephalopathy (nine days) and roughly equal to those with presumed multiple sclerosis (13 days), although the numbers were far too small to be significant.

Two patients with myasthenia gravis (Cases 38 and 39) had a dangerous but short-lived relapse a week after vaccination. This disorder is not mentioned in an authoritative list of persons who should not be vaccinated (Dixon 1962).

In a review of post-vaccinial ocular disease Rosen (1948) included the papillitis of vascular disorders such as retinal vein thrombosis and central serous retinopathy. Retrobulbar neuritis has been recorded in patients recovering from vaccinial encephalitis (Greenberg 1948, Hierons & Lyle 1959) and as an isolated sequel to vaccination (Agarwal, Dayal & Agarwal 1963).

Four days after re-vaccination in April 1967, a healthy woman aged 53 found that she could not see clearly in the passport office. Her vision previously had been excellent. Within a week she could not read the largest headlines and two months later could hardly count fingers at 1 metre. She had bilateral central scotomata and secondary optic atrophy. She did not consult her doctor for six weeks: investigations at this time included lumbar air encephalography and were all negative.

Conclusions

Experience in Cardiff in 1962 underlined the differences between post-vaccinial encephalomyelitis, with its specific histological lesion, and other types of encephalopathy and neuropathy which followed jennerian vaccination.

Vascular changes which alter capillary permeability and lower the blood-brain barrier may be important in the aetiology of the latter. Such changes are not uncommon: Rosen (1948) described post-vaccinial ocular complications due to altered capillary function and, in South Wales during 1962, Waddington and his colleagues (1964) saw 89 cases with vascular disorders of the skin (erythema, urticaria, purpura), many of them infants and small children.

Lyon, Dodge & Adams (1961) thought that the meningism of high fever predisposed to cerebral oedema and encephalopathy, no matter what the toxic agent, and Apostolov, Flewett & Thompson (1961) reported vaccinia viraemia as a cause of hyper-pyrexia and sudden infantile death. Several reviews have emphasized the special liability of infants to post-vaccinial encephalopathy and their almost total immunity to encephalomyelitis (de Vries 1960, Weber & Lange 1961, Conybeare 1964, Wilson 1967).

The viraemia of vaccinia was presumed to have caused a benign illness—meningism—in seven adults of the Cardiff series and to have precipitated three cases of encephalopathy with convulsions and three other cases of simple epilepsy. It may also have provoked relapse in six cases of multiple sclerosis and in two of myasthenia gravis. Its relation to the seven cases of peripheral nervous disorder was less obvious.

The abrupt onset, early fastigium, short period of amnesia, and uncertain pathogenesis distinguished the cases of encephalopathy from the progressive sub-cortical and spinal syndromes, and the specific histopathology, of encephalomyelitis.

REFERENCES

AGARWAL L.P., DAYAL Y. & AGARWAL P.K. (1963) Smallpox vaccination neuro-retinitis. *Orient. Arch. Ophthal.* **1**, 226–227.

APOSTOLOV K., FLEWETT T.H. & THOMPSON K.S. (1961) Death of an infant in hyperthermia after vaccination. *J. clin. Path.* **14**, 196–197.

BOUMAN L. & BOK S.T. (1927) Die Histopathologie der Encephalitis post vaccinationem. *Z. ges. Neurol. Psychiat.* **111**, 495–510.

COMBY J. (1907) L'encéphalite aiguë chez les enfants. *Archs Méd. Enf.* **10**, 577–611.

CONYBEARE E.T. (1964) Illness attributed to smallpox vaccination during 1951–1960. I. Illnesses reported as 'Generalized Vaccinia'. II. Illnesses reported as affecting the central nervous system. III. Fatal illnesses reported as associated with vaccination (but not as Generalized vaccinia or post-vaccinal encephalomyelitis). *Mon. Bull. Ministr. Hlth.* **23**, 126–133, 150–159, 182–186.

DIXON C.W. (1962) *Smallpox*. London.

GREENBERG M. (1948) Complications of vaccination against smallpox. *Amer. J. Dis. Child.* **76**, 492–502.

HIERONS R. & LYLE T.K. (1959) Bilateral retrobulbar optic neuritis. *Brain*, **82**, 56–67.

LYON G., DODGE P.R. & ADAMS R.D. (1961) The acute encephalopathies of obscure origin in infants and children. *Brain*, **84**, 680–708.

MARSDEN J.P. & HURST E.W. (1932) Acute perivascular myelinoclasis (Acute disseminated encephalomyelitis) in smallpox. *Brain*, **55**, 181–225.

PERDRAU J.R. (1928) The histology of post-vaccinal encephalitis. *J. Path. Bact.* **31**, 17–32.

ROSEN E. (1948) Postvaccinial ocular syndrome. *Amer. J. Ophthal.* **31**, 1443–1453.

SPILLANE J.D. & WELLS C.E.C. (1964) The neurology of Jennerian vaccination. A clinical account of the neurological complications which occurred during the smallpox epidemic in South Wales in 1962. *Brain*, **87**, 1–44.

TURNBULL H.M. & McINTOSH J. (1926) Encephalomyelitis following vaccination. *Br. J. exp. Path.* **7**, 181–222.

VRIES E. DE (1960) *Post-vaccinial Peri-venous Encephalitis*. Amsterdam.

WADDINGTON E., BRAY P.T., EVANS A.D. & RICHARDS I.D.G. (1964) Cutaneous complications of mass vaccination against smallpox in South Wales 1962. *Trans. St John's Hosp. derm. Soc.* **50**, 22–42.

WEBER G. & LANGE J. (1961) Zur Variationsbreite der 'Inkubationszeiten' postvakzinaler zerebraler Erkrankungen. *Dtsch. med. Wschr.* **86**, 1461–1468.

WILSON SIR G.S. (1967) *The Hazards of Immunization*. London.

Discussion of Dr Webb and Dr Wells' papers

UDALL: Dr Webb, we had a slightly different experience with the Absettarov strain of central European tick-borne encephalitis virus given to cynomolgus monkeys subcutaneously and later followed by intracerebral injection of starch, because we were interested in the production of a vaccine for louping ill. We found quite marked encephalitis at autopsy: but not particularly of the grey matter. There was damage to the dentate nuclei, the white matter of the cerebellar folia and some loss of Purkinje cells.

PALLIS: May I ask our colleagues from Compton whether they have got any information correlating the prevalence of multiple sclerosis with eating mutton or lamb? Distribution maps suggest that multiple sclerosis is common in temperate climates both north and south of the equator and rare in the tropics, where eating of mutton must be rare. Has this in fact been gone into? Also what veterinary precautions are taken to prevent Scrapie material reaching butchers' shops?

WEBB: Dr Udall, I glossed over much of the arbovirus pathology. In fact with Langat virus and KFD there is an extensive destruction in all sorts of areas of the brain. I cannot go into details. However, it always rather spoils the histology if you inoculate through the blood brain barrier. You tend to get a completely different picture from an inoculation given peripherally allowing the virus to get to the brain by whatever means it usually does. Intracerebral inoculation may give more neuronal damage.

HAIG: It has been said that multiple sclerosis is rare south of the equator and certainly that is the case with Scrapie. When it occurs it is in imported sheep. Whether or not there is any correlation between the lack of Scrapie and MS in those areas is anybody's guess. In this country Scrapie is seldom reported. The diagnosis is made by the farmer and cases are sent to slaughter before the animal loses condition and value.

DICK: I think the epidemiologists have looked carefully into the relationship of sheep and multiple sclerosis. I would like to say that histologically multiple sclerosis is nothing like Scrapie.

WATERSON: If it's any comfort to anyone there are parts of Europe especially in South Germany where mutton is not eaten at all. However, the incidence of multiple sclerosis is just the same.

HUNTER: Professor Dick, I don't think what you have just said would be true of the outer parts of the brain. There is extensive destruction of myelin with degeneration of nerve fibres and their myelin component in Scrapie, as shown by Dr Chandler and I think Dr Field.

BECK: There would be breakdown of myelin in the white matter in Scrapie or Kuru because the axons go through the white matter and the axons of the cells which are degenerating also degenerate. But it is not a primary affection of white matter as multiple sclerosis seems to be.

TOMLINSON: Is it suggested that even in acute encephalitis the real damage is done by antibody antigen interaction? Because in some of these herpes cases death has occurred before there is very much antibody. In some cases the antibody wasn't even detectable by the methods we were using. At that stage there is probably not enough viraemia to remove the antibody from the circulation. Also if it is due to antibody interaction, would not you expect some evidence from the histology?

WEBB: My point is that according to Coombs (1968) the danger arises when you have very considerable excess antigen over antibody. This allows antigen/antibody complexes to form and settle in the vessel walls and liberate other substances which produces oedema and also in my opinion the histology of the perivascular cuffing which you see. In the acute virus diseases, and possibly in multiple sclerosis, there is a concentration of lesions round vessels and the ventricular systems. I suggest that the virus is blood borne to the CNS and then spreads from cell to cell with secondary virus multiplication. This is followed by antibody production which reacts with virus at the cell surface causing enzyme release with the gross oedema one sees at post mortem. Steroids cannot do any harm at this stage and may do good by reducing cerebral oedema. If there is an antigen antibody reaction then they will be particularly good.

DICK: I was wondering, Dr Webb, whether any clinicians have tried the effect of antihistamines, not only in encephalitis but in other infections of the central nervous system.

TYRRELL: There was a study on the effects of antihistamines on virus infections of the respiratory tract. There seemed to be no detectable difference in the severity or frequency of the symptoms induced by the virus infection. This may not be entirely germane because we don't know the exact pathology of these. My own feeling however is that we don't know enough. Dr Webb's theory is very attractive but it is possible to make virus infections worse by giving cortisone and it is very difficult to decide just what stage of the disease an individual patient has reached. A deliberate controlled study of this might be valuable.

WEBB: With polio and probably with measles the encephalitic stage occurs after the end of viremia and when antibodies are present. Steroids at this stage cannot affect interferon production. There is an excellent paper by Berge (1961) and his colleagues on Venezuelan encephalitis. They gave monkeys the virus peripherally and found that if they gave cortisone only at the second fever and encephalitic stage this was very effective in damping down the abnormal histological appearances and on the survival of the animal. I think this is important.

MACCALLUM: I would like to know from some of you why do you get the picture you get in subacute sclerosing encephalitis only from the action of the measles virus or this sort of virus? Why is the lesion and the clinical picture what it is?

VAN BOGAERT: In two cases where cortisol therapy was used, especially at the stage of cerebral oedema, I thought it made them worse.

WEBB: It should be given in big doses for a very short time, and I think that the neurosurgeons will support me here, it is very useful in reducing cerebral oedema. Will someone back me up over this? I would find it difficult to do a clinical trial because for me it has worked so dramatically and I believe it can be life saving.

OPPENHEIMER: A few years ago it was current teaching that the acute perivenous and acute encephalitis associated with measles or vaccination or other infections was an immune reaction and that virus was not present in the brain in such cases. Part of the reason for believing in the immune reaction was the similarity of the histological feature to experimental allergic encephalitis. The question of virus and further infection did not come in. Is this no longer true, are viruses now demonstrated in the brains of these cases, can you tell me, Dr Webb?

WEBB: I can tell you the answer to the arboviruses, certainly yes, they are present. As regards measles I think you also have a virus. I hope Professor Waterson or Dr Tyrrell will defend me over this. Measles virus may have a tendency for multiplying in glial tissue cells. The perivenous demyelination which one sees in this disease is possibly due to multiplying virus in the glial cells which themselves produce and support myelin. I believe that demyelination is secondary to damage to the glial cells as I am convinced that myelin is produced from both astrocytes and oligodendrocytes. If the measles virus has a particular affinity for these cells for multiplication then the maximum reaction will be concentrated there and the myelin will suffer as a result. The reaction is determined by the site of multiplication. Measles virus is notoriously difficult to detect whereas the arbovirus is easy.

LEGG: I don't say I agree with Dr Webb about the usefulness of steroids, but in looking through the literature and talking to clinicians I have not found any disasters from giving steroids with encephalitis. This may be because the interferon stage has passed by that time. Disasters recorded, either experimentally or clinically, are with steroids given at the time of the original infection. Dr Webb's view of the pathogenesis of encephalitis is much more questionable; and we should not be dogmatic about steroids. They may work simply by their action on any form of cerebral oedema. Presumably they have not been shown to have any effect in subacute sclerosing panencephalitis, because, although there is a possibility that this is some form of neuro-allergic encephalitis, they don't suppress antibody formation or whatever reaction is going on in the brain.

CHAIRMAN: I think we must close this discussion now.

Viruses, Malignant Disease and the Nervous System

Chairman
S. Nevin

Viruses, Malignant Disease and the Nervous System

A.P.Waterson and June D.Almeida

Tumours, both benign and malignant, can be caused by a wide range of aetiological factors, from ionizing radiations and chemical carcinogens to viruses. It is not at all surprising that viruses should give rise to neoplasms, as we now appreciate that viruses can do several things to cells other than kill them. Ever since the transmission by Peyton Rous in 1911 of a sarcoma of fowls 'by an agent separable from the tumor cells', the fact of viral oncogenesis has been established beyond doubt, and there is a large array of neoplastic conditions (including leukaemias) known to be caused by viruses (Gross 1961) and occurring in several species of vertebrate (Table 14).

The property of oncogenicity, i.e. the ability to cause tumours, is not limited to a single morphological type of virus. On the contrary, while some tumours are identical in form with non-oncogenic viruses, e.g. those of the adenovirus group (Figs. 49a, b) others have a distinctive morphology which has not yet been recognized among non-oncogenic viruses, e.g. the virus (Fig. 50) of the Bittner mouse mammary carcinoma (Almeida, Waterson & Drewe 1967). The term 'tumour virus', or 'oncogenic virus', can therefore be used only in the widest sense, i.e. to indicate a virus which has, in some host, under some conditions, caused a tumour. The term, in fact, embraces a wide range of viruses united by the one property of oncogenicity, but perhaps widely separated in the means they use to achieve this result.

The oncogenic potential of a virus may have to be sought diligently before it is revealed, and it is probably not too much to say that, given the correct conditions, any virus may prove to be a tumour virus. The hallmark of an oncogenic virus is that it interacts with a cell in such a way that the cell is altered but not killed, otherwise a descendant line of malignant cells would not arise. Viruses seem to produce malignant change in one of two ways, depending on the type of viral nucleic acid. RNA viruses seem to enter into a kind of symbiotic arrangement with the cell which results in malignant transformation of the cell, but at the same time allows virus production to proceed. On the other hand DNA viruses appear to be incorporated, at least in part, into the

TABLE 14. Some common oncogenic viruses of vertebrates

Natural host	Tumour host	Virus	Neoplasm	Nucleic acid	Symmetry	Type of morphology
mouse	mouse	leukaemia (Gross)	leukaemia	RNA	unknown	unknown
—	hamster	polyoma	various	DNA	cubic	polyoma-wart group
—	mouse	Bittner	mammary carcinoma	RNA	unknown	spherical capsid, with envelope
rabbit	rabbit	Shope papilloma	papilloma or carcinoma of skin	DNA	cubic	polyoma-wart group
—	rabbit	Shope fibroma	fibroma	DNA	poxvirus	poxvirus
fowl	fowl	Rous	sarcoma	RNA	unknown	unknown
—	fowl	avian erythromyeloblastosis	erythromyeloblastosis	RNA	helical	compound helical RNA
—	fowl	neurolymphomatosis	Marek's disease (neurolymphomatosis)	DNA	cubic	herpes group
frog	frog	Lucké	adenoma or adeno-carcinoma	DNA	cubic	herpes group
man	hamster	some adenoviruses (e.g. type 12)	sarcoma	DNA	cubic	adenovirus

genome of the cell, as revealed by the production of virally coded T-antigens in the transformed cell. That it is only a partial incorporation is suggested by the fact that the classical methods of induction effective for bacteriophages fail to reveal an unexpressed virus.

It would be surprising if man, with the wide variety of tumours found in all systems of his body, does not, like other vertebrates which have been studied, have at least some tumours which can be transmitted by viruses, and are caused by them, either alone or in association with other factors. Unfortunately for those favouring viruses as a main cause of tumours, no malignant tumour of man, and only one benign human tumour (the common wart), is known to be caused by a virus. However, there are a few situations in human medicine where viruses are found in situations whose relevance to neoplasia merits examination (see Table 15).

1   *The common wart*, (Fig. 48) whose virus is found in large quantities in the cells of warts. It is a DNA cubic virus, size 550 Å, which has not yet been grown *in vitro*.

2   *Molluscum contagiosum*. This infective condition of the skin is caused by a member of the poxvirus group (Fig. 51). Although the lesions bear some resemblance macroscopically to benign tumours, they are not histologically neoplastic, and always regress spontaneously.

3   *Burkitt's lymphoma*. Of the several viruses isolated from this malignant tumour, most are almost certainly 'passengers', but one of them (the EB, or Epstein-Barr) virus does at least merit consideration as a possible aetiological agent. It is morphologically typical of the herpes group, and can be studied in cultured cells of the tumour, but has not been produced *in vitro* apart from them.

4   *Progressive multifocal leuco-encephalopathy* (*PML*). In this condition, which occurs in association chiefly with reticuloses such as Hodgkin's disease or chronic lymphatic leukaemia, particles of a virus morphologically similar to mouse polyoma virus (Fig. 47) are found in the nuclei of oligodendrocytes (Zu Rhein 1967). Its role in the aetiology both of the PML and of the tumour is unknown. However, viruses, like man, are known by the company they keep, and any virus which consorts (albeit morphologically) with polyoma and SV40 viruses, puts itself in a very compromising position. It has not been grown *in vitro*.

In addition to these four conditions, several adenoviruses isolated from man are oncogenic if injected into newborn hamsters, but it must be emphasized that there is no evidence that they are oncogenic in man.

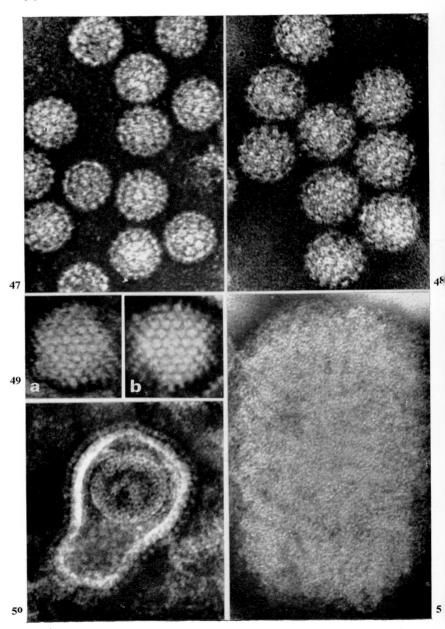

When the specific question of the connection between viruses, cancer, and the central nervous system is considered, it must be conceded that there is no more, and no less, evidence for viruses as causes of tumours in the CNS than in other systems. Polyoma virus injected into the brains of hamsters and other rodents has sometimes been followed by tumours of the meninges, but more frequently by hydrocephalus secondary to inflammation around the aqueduct of Sylvius. Nevertheless there are other and more subtle points of contact between virology. neurology and cancer:

1   *Carcinomatous neuropathies.* It has been suggested that some of these syndromes, occurring within the CNS in association with malignancy outside it, may be caused by viruses, and in the case of PML this seems probable. It is also possible that the virus may have caused the neoplastic condition as well as the neuropathy.

2   *Chronic progressive disorders of the CNS.* Some of these, e.g. motor neurone disease, occur in association with malignant disease and are here ranked as carcinomatous neuropathies, but principally they occur apart from any known neoplasia. If it should be proved that they are due to a virus when occurring in association with neoplasms, they may also be expected to be caused by a virus when occurring apart from neoplasms.

3   *Slow virus infections of the CNS.* Finally it might be worth considering the possibility that the pathology of slow infections of the CNS may occupy a position not too far removed from the viral oncogenesis which we have been considering. The slow infection of the human CNS about which most is known virologically is subacute sclerosing panencephalitis (SSPE), the causative organism of which is almost certainly measles (Symposium 1968). Since measles is an RNA virus this condition invites comparison with known oncogenic RNA viruses. Bittner virus infects C3H mice immediately after birth, via the mother's milk, but the mice do not develop mammary tumours till some 18 months

---

All figures are electron micrographs of virus particles prepared by the negative staining technique, using phosphotungstic acid. The magnification is × 300,000.

FIGURE 47. Polyoma virus.
FIGURE 48. Human common wart virus.
FIGURE 49. Adenoviruses. (a) Type 5. (b) Type 12. Type 12 is known to be oncogenic in hamsters.
FIGURE 50. Bittner mouse mammary carcinoma virus.
FIGURE 51. Molluscum contagiosum virus.

TABLE 15. Human neoplastic and other conditions associated with viruses

Lesion	Status	Proved viral aetiology	Virus	Nature	Growth of virus in cell culture
Common wart	Benign neoplasm	+	Wart virus	DNA virus with cubic symmetry. Size 550 Å. Morphologically typical of polyoma-wart group	−
Molluscum contagiosum	Regresses naturally Not histologically neoplastic	+	Molluscum contagiosum virus	DNA virus; morphologically a poxvirus	−
Progressive multifocal leucoencephalopathy (PML)	Neuropathy occurring in association with certain reticuloses and malignant tumours	?	PML virus	Morphologically identical with polyoma and SV40 viruses. Size 450 Å	−
Burkitt lymphoma	Malignant neoplasm	?	EB (Epstein-Barr) virus	Morphologically a herpesvirus	±

later. The various mouse leukaemia viruses have average latent periods of around eight months. With almost all artificially transferred onco-genic viruses the age of the donor is critical, as the efficiency of produc-tion of tumours drops sharply in mice infected when over 48 hours old. There is in these facts, i.e. in the relation between latent period and age of infection, a similarity to the course of SSPE. In both situations there is a prolonged latent period during which virus is undetectable. At the end of this time virus once again appears, and in the case of the RNA oncogenic viruses this is accompanied by neoplastic change. In the case of SSPE, while the principal changes are destructive, there is nevertheless a proliferation of astrocytes. The resemblance is sufficient to warrant a closer look at the possibility that the virus in SSPE re-sembles an oncogenic RNA virus more closely than it does the more orthodox necrotizing type.

In SSPE the virus seems to remain latent only in the CNS, and this could suggest that the virus retained in latent form is itself deficient in some way and requires some special circumstance of the CNS to allow its continuance in this form. It is noteworthy that the amount of measles viral ribonucleoprotein present in the brain in SSPE far exceeds that of complete virus, and indeed represents virtually all the morpho-logically identifiable virus seen.

To sum up, slow viruses infecting the CNS appear to resemble certain oncogenic viruses by reason of their long latent period and the need to enter a susceptible organism at an early age. They differ from oncogenic viruses in that they do not initiate a neoplastic response, but nevertheless seem to stimulate a proliferative one. However, in terms of their molecular biology (rather than their final and overall clinical effect in the host) infections by all of the viruses which we have been considering may be variations upon a common theme, whose original form is embodied in the lysogenic bacterium.

REFERENCES

ALMEIDA J.D., WATERSON A.P. & DREWE J.A. (1967) A morphological comparison of Bittner and influenza viruses. *J. Hyg. (Camb.)*, **65**, 467–474.

GROSS L. (1961) *Oncogenic Viruses*. Oxford.

SYMPOSIUM ON SUBACUTE SCLEROSING PANENCEPHALITIS (1968) *Neurology (Minneap.)*, **18**, 1–192.

ZU RHEIN G.M. (1967) Polyoma-like virions in a human demyelinating disease. *Acta neuropathologica*, **8**, 57–68.

Progressive Multifocal Leukoencephalopathy

A. D. Dayan

Identification and preliminary characterization of a new disease often depend on both clinical and morbid anatomical observations. It is fortunate that such findings may sometimes be so striking that they suggest a possible aetiology which can then be further investigated by more refined techniques.

Amongst recently recognized disorders of the nervous system are two which have been clarified by the sequential application of these processes—Subacute Sclerosing Panencephalitis which may be caused by measles virus (Symposium 1968), and Progressive Multifocal Leukoencephalopathy (PML) which appears to be due to infection of the brain by a polyoma-like virus (Silverman & Rubinstein 1965, Woodhouse, Dayan, Burston, Caldwell, Melcher, Adams & Urich 1967).

Clinical features of PML

Richardson (1961, 1965) has summarized the clinical presentation of PML as a rapidly progressive, relentless disorder of the central nervous system in which widespread dissemination of lesions accounts for the divers symptoms and signs. Most reports have been of patients aged 30 to 60 years, who have suffered for a few weeks to a few months from a variety of dementia, pareses, visual field defects, ataxias, etc. There are almost twice as many reports of men with PML as women (Richardson 1965, Sloof, 1966, ZuRhein 1967). Unusual clinical forms of the disease have included cases with a very slow progression, some-times lasting for many years (Stam 1966, Hedley-Whyte, Smith, Tyler & Peterson 1966), and two with a peripheral neuropathy (Fisher, Williams & Wing 1960, Sadka 1963).

Almost all cases of PML have occurred in patients who were already suffering from a lymphoma or some other disorder of the reticulo-endothelial system. The association, which was noted in the first account of PML (Aström, Mancall & Richardson 1958) has been confirmed by the majority of subsequent reports.

Pathology. In brains affected by PML typically there are widely disseminated small round greyish areas at the junction of the grey and white matter of the cerebral cortex. However, lesions occur anywhere in the central nervous system and sometimes are very extensive (Richardson 1965). There are no characteristic findings in the systemic tissues of patients suffering from PML.

The striking histological features of PML led to the first hypotheses about its aetiology. There are foci of true demyelination (Fig. 52) with relative sparing of axis cylinders. Glial cells in affected areas

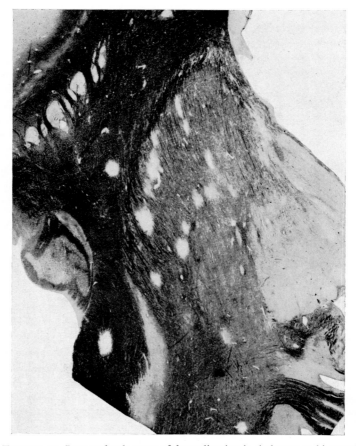

FIGURE 52. Scattered pale areas of demyelination in thalamus and internal capsule of a case of progressive multifocal leukoencephalopathy (Luxol fast blue, ×4·5).

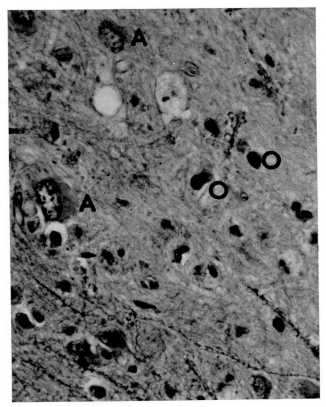

FIGURE 53. Edge of a lesion showing abnormal astrocytes (A) and enlarged hyperchromatic oligodendrocyte nuclei (O) (Klüver-Barrera, × 100).

usually show two characteristic changes (Fig. 53). Some astrocytes become greatly enlarged and have bizarre, distorted nuclei. Abnormal mitoses may sometimes be seen in such cells. Lesions also contain more typical appearing hypertrophic astrocytes. In the centres of smaller foci and around the rims of larger ones many oligodendroglial nuclei appear abnormally large and deeply basophilic, and in some amphophilic or basophilic inclusions may be seen.

Hypotheses about the aetiology of PML

The striking association between lesions of cerebral white matter, particularly the type of damage to oligodendroglia, and disorders of the reticulo-endothelial system led to suggestions that it might be due to an auto-immune reaction against the brain, or to an opportunistic viral infection of the nervous system in patients whose immune defences had been damaged by the primary disease (Aström *et al.* 1958, Cavanagh, Greenbaum, Marshall & Rubinstein 1959, Richardson 1965). Because of the intranuclear inclusions and other features suggesting a viral infection, brains from cases of PML have recently been examined by several physical and biological techniques.

Electron microscopy of the brain in PML

Virus-like particles were reported independently in 1965 in brains from five cases of PML by Silverman & Rubinstein, Vanderhaeghen & Perier, and by Howatson, Nagai & ZuRhein. Similar observations have since been made by Woodhouse *et al.* (1967), and ZuRhein (1967), and the total number of cases successfully examined by electron microscopy is now more than twenty.

In all the brains there have been similar findings in abnormal glial nuclei, probably of oligodendrocytes, of many rounded or filamentous virus-like particles sometimes forming geometrical arrays (Figs. 54, 55). In thin sections the round particles have had diameters of 350–450 Å. Howatson *et al.* (1965) isolated the particles, and showed in negatively stained preparations that they had diameters of about 410 Å, and that their surfaces were studded with complex projections like capsomeres.

Further evidence about the physical nature of the particles in an unfixed, autopsy sample of brain from one case of PML was obtained by Schwerdt, Schwerdt, Silverman & Rubinstein (1966). They showed that the particles had a density of about 1·30–1·31 on equilibrium centrifugation of a partly purified homogenate in caesium chloride. On negative staining of this fraction, round particles were seen, 380 Å in diameter, with 16 or 17 capsomeres around their peripheries separated by about 7–8 Å. Schwerdt *et al.* inoculated some of the brain onto monolayer cultures of several human tissues including glial cells, and they injected aliquots into new-born hamsters. No evidence of a transmitted infection was obtained in any of the biological experiments.

Conclusions about the aetiology of PML

The clinical associations and pathological features of PML suggest that it might be due to an unusual viral infection of the central nervous system. Electron microscopy has shown that there are intranuclear

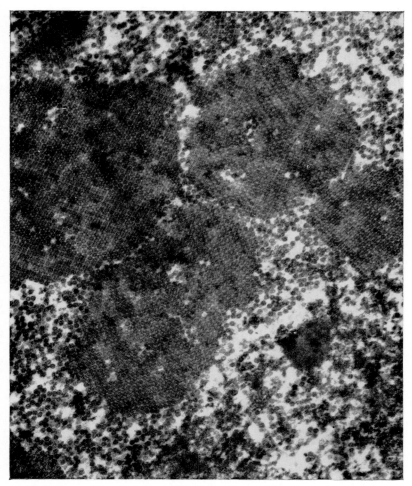

FIGURE 54. Round virus particles lying free and in geometric arrays in nucleus of a glial cell (× 36,000).

particles in glial cells which have many of the morphological and physical features of a "virus" belonging to the papova group (Melnick 1962), and most closely resembling polyoma virus. The evidence so far is almost entirely based on morphology as the more rigid methods of classical virology have still to be applied, to PML. It is disturbing that the reported sizes of particles isolated from brains of PML patients

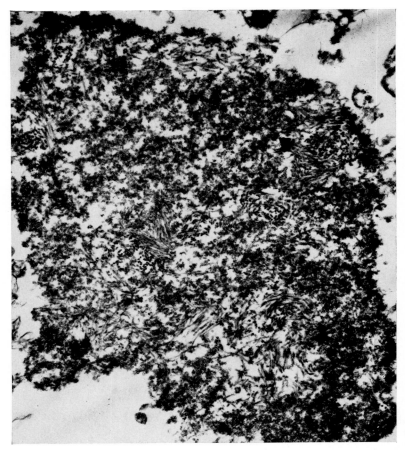

FIGURE 55. Filamentous virus particles in a glial cell nucleus (× 18,000).

have been so varied but this may be due to the largely unstudied effects on viruses of fixation and processing of tissues for sectioning, failure to allow for the geometric distortion of measurements made on spherical objects of a diameter comparable to the thickness of the section in which they lie (Abercrombie 1946), and other difficulties discussed by Almeida, Waterson & Fletcher (1966). At present, apart from size, further difficulties in accepting the virus as polyoma are that in experimental infections in animals it is not known to cause damage to the nervous system like PML (summarized by Woodhouse *et al.* 1967, and ZuRhein 1967); no positive serological evidence of its identity has been obtained, and that Schwerdt *et al.* were unable to grow virus in preparations usually considered suitable for polyoma. However, the histological appearances of bizarre astrocytes in PML are reminiscent of cells transformed by this virus (Howatson *et al.*) and the negatively-stained and thin section electron micrographs are strongly suggestive of polyoma.

Only one of Koch's postulates has been fulfilled so far, but the morphological evidence available suggests that PML is probably due to infection of the nervous system by a virus which may best be considered as polyoma-like. Further investigations are required to decide whether it is polyoma or some related but hitherto undescribed virus, and to examine the nature of its unusual effect on the nervous system of causing demyelination.

REFERENCES

ABERCROMBIE M. (1946) Estimation of nuclear population from microtome sections. *Anat. Rec.* **94**, 239–247.

ALMEIDA J.D., WATERSON A.P. & FLETCHER W.L. (1966) Interpretation of structural detail in viruses of the polyoma group. *Progr. Exp. Tumour Res.* **8**, 95–124.

ASTRÖM K.E., MANCALL E.L. & RICHARDSON E.P. (1958) Progressive multifocal leukoencephalopathy. *Brain*, **81**, 93–111.

CAVANAGH J.B., GREENBAUM D., MARSHALL A.H.E. & RUBINSTEIN L.J. (1959) Cerebral demyelination associated with disorders of the reticulo-endothelial system. *Lancet*, ii, 524–529.

FISHER C.M., WILLIAMS H.W. & WING E.S. (1960) Combined encephalopathy and neuropathy with carcinoma. *J. Neuropathol. Exp. Neurol.* **20**, 535–547.

HEDLEY-WHYTE E.T., SMITH B.P., TYLER H.R. & PATERSON W.P. (1966) Multifocal leukoencephalopathy with remission and five year survival. *J. Neuropathol. Exp. Neurol.* **25**, 107–116.

HOWATSON, A.F., NAGAI M. & ZuRHEIN G.M. (1965) Polyoma-like virions in human demyelinating brain disease. *Canad. Med. Assoc. J.* **93**, 379–386.

MELNICK J.L. (1962) Papova virus group. *Science*, **135**, 1128–1130.

RICHARDSON E.P. (1961) Progressive multifocal leukoencephalopathy. *New Engl. J. Med.* **265**, 815–823.

RICHARDSON E.P. (1965) Progressive multifocal leukoencephalopathy. In *Remote Effects of Cancer on the Nervous System*, W.R. Brain & F.H. Norris (ed.) New York, p. 6.

SADKA M. (1963) Progressive multifocal leukoencephalopathy. *Proc. Austral. Assoc. Neurol.* **1**, 13–17.

SCHWERDT P.R., SCHWERDT C.E., SILVERMAN L. & RUBINSTEIN L.J. (1966) Virions associated with progressive multifocal leukoencephalopathy. *Virol.* **29**, 511–514.

SILVERMAN L. & RUBINSTEIN L.J. (1965) Electron microscopic observations on a case of progressive multifocal leukoencephalopathy. *Acta. Neuropathol. (Berl.)* **5**, 215–224.

SLOOF J.L. (1966) Two cases of progressive multifocal leukoencephalopathy with unusual aspects. *Psychiat. Neurol. Neurochir.* **69**, 461–474.

STAM F.C. (1966) Multifocal leukoencephalopathy with slow progression and long survival. *Psychiat. Neurol. Neurochir.* **69**, 453–459.

SYMPOSIUM (1968) Measles virus and subacute sclerosing panencephalitis. *Neurol. (Minneap.),* **18**, No. 1, pt. 2.

VANDERHAEGHEN J.J. & PERIER O. (1965) Leuco-encéphalite multifocale progressive. *Acta Neurol. Psychiat. Belg.* **65**, 816–836.

WOODHOUSE M.A., DAYAN A.D., BURSTON J., CALDWELL I., MELCHER D., ADAMS J.H. & URICH H. (1967) Progressive multifocal leukoencephalopathy: electron microscope study of four cases. *Brain*, **90**, 863–870.

ZuRHEIN G.M. (1967) Polyoma-like virions in a human demyelinating disease. *Acta Neuropathol. (Berl.),* **8**, 57–68.

Sub-acute Encephalitis and Malignancy

J. A. N. Corsellis

A variety of neurological disorders have been identified in the last few years which may occur in association with carcinoma. Professor Urich will be discussing the neuropathological aspects of these conditions in some detail. Briefly, however, the main histological findings consist of neuronal loss, a glial reaction, and possibly some tract degeneration, occurring in the hind-brain and spinal cord. There may also be histological evidence of an inflammatory reaction which can at times be so severe as to be indistinguishable from that seen in viral encephalitis.

Until recently these 'inflammatory' changes were thought to be restricted to levels caudal to the basal ganglia. There is now evidence, however, that they may also occur on some occasions within the cerebral hemispheres but with particular emphasis on the limbic areas. When this happens, moreover, the patients may develop disturbance of memory or become demented.

The first patient in which this condition was described appears to be one reported in 1960 by Brierley, Corsellis, Hierons & Nevin in their study of several cases of an obscure encephalitis lasting a few months and occurring in late adult life. The main pathological feature was the way in which the inflammatory reaction was concentrated in the limbic areas of the cerebral mantle. One of these patients was a man of 58 who deteriorated mentally for no known reason. After death a severe 'limbic' encephalitis was identified; the only other pathological abnormality was secondary carcinomatous deposits in the mediastinal lymph nodes. At the time of this report the evidence linking an inflammatory reaction in the brain to the presence of a bronchial carcinoma seemed too tenuous to justify the suggestion of anything other than coincidence.

The following year Verhaart (1961) described degeneration of the cerebral grey matter in a man of 51 who had developed a psychiatric illness of an inorganic type and in whom after death mediastinal lymph nodes were found to contain secondary carcinomatous deposits. Verhaart placed particular emphasis on the macroscopic discolouration of both hippocampi which he found was due to a degenerative process concentrated in these areas and in the surrounding grey matter. The brain stem was also slightly affected.

The next report was made by Störring, Hauss & Ule (1962) in an article discussing the cerebral localization of memory disturbance. They described the clinical and pathological findings in a man of 49 who developed a severe loss of memory during the course of a fatal illness resulting from carcinoma of the bronchus. Again the unusually dark colour of the hippocampal grey matter was emphasized, while the histological picture was that of an inflammatory reaction mainly affecting the limbic grey matter.

Three years later a further report appeared by Yahr, Duvoisin & Cowen (1965). The patient was a woman of 61 with a 12 months' history of psychiatric disorder which included a severe defect of recent memory. No macroscopic abnormality was seen in the brain. Histologically, however, the 'limbic' areas were again found to be the region chiefly involved in what the authors felt was a degenerative rather than an inflammatory process, although in the published discussion of their paper they agreed that the findings could be interpreted as the effect of a viral infection.

Still more recently, Ulrich, Spiess & Huber (1967) have reported yet another example of an organic psychiatric illness occurring in the presence of a bronchial carcinoma. Once again the cerebral damage was concentrated on the temporal component of the limbic areas, and in particular on the hippocampi in which there was evidence of considerable degeneration as well as an inflammatory reaction.

With the previous reports in mind, three further examples may now be summarized. The first was a bus driver, who at the age of 59 suffered several convulsive attacks, followed a few weeks later by the sudden onset of a marked and permanent loss of recent memory, for which no cause was found. Until his death two years later the patient continued to have an occasional epileptic attack, but there was little or no intellectual deterioration during this time. On questioning he remembered his former bus routes in detail, but although he could register new information he could not recall it two to three minutes later. The possibility of a subacute encephalitis affecting the temporal lobes, or of secondary deposits in these areas, was considered, but no primary growth was identified. After his death, however, an enlarged mediastinal lymph node was found to have been infiltrated by cells similar to those seen in an oat-celled bronchial carcinoma.

In the brain the hippocampi and the subicular cortex on both sides showed a brownish discolouration easily seen by the naked eye. Histologically, mild cuffing of a few small vessels was scattered throughout the brain, but the severe damage was focused on the medial temporal areas. Here there was an extensive loss of nerve cells, with marked proliferation of astrocytes and fibrous gliosis; perivascular infiltration by small round cells was also present. The right amygdaloid nucleus contained a small patch of necrosis. The subiculum and the Ammon's horn on both sides were severely damaged, and the degeneration extended throughout the length of both fornices, the anterior columns being heavily gliosed in their course through the hypothalamus. Both mamillary bodies showed neuronal loss, glial proliferation, and a few glial nodules.

The second case was a man of 50 known to be suffering from a carcinoma of the lung, who became mildly demented with some disorientation and impairment of recent memory. The lower lobe of his left lung was resected and was found to contain a bronchial carcinoma. The mental state of the patient showed little post-operative change, but he gradually developed dysarthria and the weakness and wasting of the small muscles of his limbs, which had been noted before the operation, became worse. He died after an illness lasting about two years. After death no evidence of a recurrence of the intra-thoracic growth was found.

Histological examination of the brain revealed mild patchy cuffing of small vessels in the leptomeninges, most noticeable over the cingular gyrus but also seen at rare intervals over the rest of the hemispheres. Perivascular cuffing was found in and around the amygdaloid nucleus, in the anterior cingular cortex, along the border of the third ventricle, in the hypothalamus and adjacent to the caudate nucleus. The tectum of the mid-brain, the pons and medulla also showed some cuffing of vessels. The amygdaloid nucleus, parahippocampal gyrus, substantia nigra, and the inferior olives contained small well-packed aggregations of glial nuclei, often apparently encircling necrotic nerve cells. Glial stars were also seen between the thalamus and the lining of the third ventricle.

The third case was a woman of 81 who died after a psychiatric illness lasting some years and marked in its later stages by dementia and a severe defect of recent memory. Malignant disease had not been suspected during life, but after death the main bronchi of both lungs and the adjacent mediastinal lymph nodes were found to be infiltrated by an oat-celled carcinoma.

Histological examination of the brain showed the medial temporal areas to have been severely damaged; there were numerous glial nodules, diffuse astrocytic proliferation with fibrous gliosis, and a moderate loss of nerve cells, particularly in the subiculum, while the small vessels in these areas showed lymphocytic cuffing. The mid-brain, substantia nigra, and the pons and medulla also showed some glial nodules and an occasional cuffed vessel.

Discussion

The reports and cases that have been brought together here suggest that the occurrence of a 'limbic encephalitis' in some patients with carcinoma, and particularly with bronchial carcinoma, is more than coincidence.

When the patients in these various reports are considered as a group, the clinical histories are seen to have had some features in common. A marked disturbance of affect was usual. With one possible exception a striking feature was a disorder of recent memory, and some degree of dementia was usually, but not always, found. Several patients had suffered epileptic attacks. A few had shown evidence of a carcinomatous neuromyopathy.

The cerebro-spinal fluid was abnormal in all but one of the seven cases in which it was examined, the abnormality being a raised lympho-cyte count and/or a raised protein level.

Electro-encephalographic records had been made in four of the patients and all were abnormal, the abnormalities tending to be most marked over the temporal lobes.

On the pathological side the most remarkable feature was the concen-tration of the microscopic and, in several cases, the macroscopic changes in the medial parts of the grey matter of the temporal lobes.

Whether these changes should be considered as inflammatory or degenerative is not at present clear and will presumably remain a problem until their cause is known. Although the relative severity of the inflammatory component has varied greatly from case to case, it has at times been severe enough to be indistinguishable from a viral encephalitis Indeed, some workers (Henson, Hoffman & Urich 1965) have suggested that the condition may be the result of a viral infection, and Dayan, Bhatti & Gostling (1967) have recently mentioned the herpes simplex virus in this connection, partly because of the way in which the pathological damage tends to focus on the temporal lobes. There are, however, noticeable differences between the herpetic and the carcinomatous forms of encephalitis. In the former the illness is usually acute and the damage is massive, with gross destruction of tissue spreading beyond the limbic areas into the temporal lobes and even further. In the patients with carcinoma and 'limbic encephalitis' the illness is insidious, and the pathological process is less widespread and much less severe. There is also the fact that, apart from the case reported by Dayan and his colleagues, intra-nuclear inclusion bodies have not been demonstrated in association with the carcinomatous form.

Lastly it is conceivable that not all cases of acute and subacute necrotizing encephalitis affecting the temporal lobes are due to an infection with the herpes simplex virus. The present speaker has seen one typical sub-acute example in which the organism isolated from the patient's cerebro-spinal fluid was the Coxsackie B5 virus (Heathfield, Pilsworth, Wall & Corsellis 1967). Several other unpublished examples of obscure aetiology include one which followed immediately after anti-venom treatment for snake-bite.

It seems therefore premature to incriminate the herpes simplex virus as a cause of the tissue reaction in these cases although no other more satisfactory explanation appears to be forthcoming, viral, metabolic and immune factors all being easier to invoke than to verify.

Finally, no hypothesis is known to the present speaker which would adequately explain the remarkable way in which the pathological process in these cases tends to focus on the limbic grey matter and in particular on its temporal component.

This paper is an abbreviated version of a more detailed report entitled 'Limbic Encephalitis and its Association with Carcinoma' (Corsellis, Goldberg & Norton (1968) *Brain*, **91**, 481–496).

REFERENCES

BRIERLEY J.B., CORSELLIS J.A.N., HIERONS R. & NEVIN S. (1960) Subacute encephalitis of later adult life. *Brain*, **83**, 357–368.

CORSELLIS J.A.N., GOLDBERG G.J. & NORTON A.R. (1968) 'Limbic encephalitis' and its association with carcinoma. *Brain*, **91**, 481–496.

DAYAN A.D., BHATTI I. & GOSTLING J.V.T. (1967) Encephalitis due to herpes simplex in a patient with treated carcinoma of uterus. *Neurology, Minneap.* **17**, 609–613.

HEATHFIELD K.W.G., PILSWORTH R., WALL B.J. & CORSELLIS J.A.N. (1967) Coxsackie B5 infections with particular reference to the nervous system. *Quart. J. Med.* **36**, 579–595.

HENSON R. A., HOFFMAN H. L. & URICH H. (1965) Encephalomyelitis with carcinoma. *Brain*, **88**, 449–464.

STÖRRING G. E., HAUSS K. & ULE G. (1962) On the topical diagnosis of the amnesic symptom complex. *Psychiat. et Neurol.* (*Basel*), **143**, 161–177.

ULRICH J., SPIESS H. & HUBER R. (1967) Neurological syndromes as a distant effect of malignant tumour. *Schweiz. Arch. Neurol. Neurochir. Psychiat.* **99**, 83–100.

VERHAART W. J. C. (1961) Grey matter degeneration of the central nervous system in carcinosis. *Acta Neuropath.* (*Berl.*), **1**, 107–112.

YAHR M. D., DUVOISIN R. C. & COWEN D. (1965) Encephalopathy associated with carcinoma. *Trans. Amer. neurol. Ass.* **90**, 80–86.

The Neurological Syndromes Associated with Carcinoma

Marcia Wilkinson

The neurological syndromes associated with carcinoma are many and varied, but only those possibly associated with virus infections of the nervous system will be dealt with in any detail here. The work described was based on a study organized by the late Lord Brain and financed by the British Empire Cancer Campaign. Dr Peter Croft and I have done the clinical studies. We are most grateful to the physicians and surgeons of The London Hospital and to our colleagues elsewhere for allowing us to study their patients.

It is only within the last twenty years that the various clinical syndromes due to the remote effects of cancer on the nervous system have been fully described although some reference was made to them as early as 1890 by Auché. In 1948 Denny-Brown described the sensory neuropathies, in 1950 Lennox and Pritchard the peripheral neuropathies and in the following year Brain, Daniel & Greenfield reported the association of carcinoma and subacute cerebellar degeneration. Since this time the literature on the subject has grown rapidly and with it our knowledge of the clinical syndromes which may occur and of the underlying pathological changes. The actual mechanism or mechanisms by which these syndromes are produced is still uncertain. Over 100,000 patients die each year from malignant tumours and from our figures it seems probable that 6% of these have some evidence of carcinomatous neuromyopathy. This means that at any one time approximately 6000 people in the United Kingdom will have clinical signs of carcinomatous neuromyopathy. 17,000 patients die each year from carcinoma of the bronchus and our figures suggest that 2500 of these will probably have evidence of neuromyopathy.

Till a short time ago very little attempt had been made to make a classification of the types and sites of the neurological disorders which might occur with neoplasm. A Symposium was held in Rochester in October 1964 and following this Brain & Adams (1965) put forward a new classification of the carcinomatous neuromyopathies. They divided these into the following groups.

213

The encephalopathies

1 Multifocal leucoencephalopathy
2 Diffuse polioencephalopathy
   (a) With mental symptoms
   (b) With subacute cerebellar degeneration
   (c) With brain-stem lesions
3 Encephalopathies due to disordered metabolic or endocrine functions or nutritional deficiency, especially:
   (a) Hypercalcaemia with or without metastases
   (b) Hyperadrenalism
   (c) Hypoglycaemia
   (d) Hyponatraemia or water intoxication
   (e) Hyperviscosity states especially in macroglobulinaemia

The myelopathies

1 Chronic myelopathy
   (a) With long tract degeneration
   (b) With long tract and neuronal degeneration
   (c) Cases simulating motor neurone disease
2 Subacute necrotic myelopathy
3 Nutritional myelopathy

The neuropathies

1 Sensory neuropathy with dorsal column degeneration
2 Peripheral sensorimotor neuropathy (polyneuropathy or polyneuritis)
3 Metabolic, endocrine and nutritional neuropathy

The muscular disorders

1 Polymyopathy
2 Disorders of muscular transmission
   (a) Myasthenic myopathy with paradoxical potentiation
   (b) Myasthenia gravis
3 Polymyositis and dermatomyositis
4 Metabolic myopathies secondary to disordered endocrine function, especially:
   (a) Hyperadrenalism
   (b) Hypercalcaemia
   (c) Hyperthyroidism

These types may all appear singly or in combination.

It seems possible that the remote effects of cancer on the central nervous system may well be associated with virus infection. This is probably so in the case of progressive multifocal leucoencephalopathy, and also in the encephalitis-ganglioradiculitis range of disorders. It may apply, too, to the cord lesions such as the motor neurone type and subacute necrotic myelopathy, but we have no definite pathological evidence of this at present. It seems improbable that virus infections play any part in the peripheral sensorimotor neuropathies or the myopathies unless a subclinical virus infection renders the host more likely to develop these syndromes.

TABLE 16. Incidence of carcinomatous neuromyopathy

| | Survey | | | |
| | No. of | Neuromyopathy | | Selected |
Site of growth	patients	No.	%	cases
Breast	250	11	4·4	7
Lung	316	45	14·2	40
Stomach	178	16	9·0	1
Colon	160	6	3·8	1
Rectum	207	1	0·5	1
Ovary	55	9	16·4	2
Cervix	144	3	2·1	—
Uterus	76	1	1·3	1
Prostate	31	2	6·4	1
Multiple primaries	48	2	4·2	1
Miscellaneous primaries	—	—	—	11
Total	1465	96	6·6	66

A series of 1465 patients with carcinoma was examined and in addition any patients who were referred because they were thought to have a neuromyopathy. The incidence in the group as a whole was just over 6% (Croft & Wilkinson 1965). Table 16 shows the number of patients examined, the site of the primary cancer and the incidence of neuromyopathy in the series. The incidence is highest in patients with carcinoma of the lung, ovary and stomach and lowest in those with carcinoma of the rectum, cervix and uterus.

Table 17 gives the incidence of the different types of neuromyopathy. The abnormality most commonly found is that called a 'neuromuscular

TABLE 17. The incidence of some different types of carcinomatous neuromyopathy seen in routine examination of patients with carcinoma, and in selected patients referred because of evidence of neuromyopathy

Patients	Type of neuromyopathy*							Total
	Cerebellar degeneration	Myelopathy	Motor neurone type	Sensory neuropathy	Mixed peripheral neuropathy	Myopathy including myasthenia	Neuro-muscular	
Series	3 (3%)	3 (3%)	3 (3%)	—	18 (19%)	15 (16%)	62 (65%)	96
Selected	12 (18%)	12 (18%)	8 (12%)	8 (12%)	18 (27%)	11 (17%)	15 (23%)	66
All patients	15 (9%)	15 (9%)	11 (7%)	8 (5%)	36 (22%)	26 (16%)	77 (48%)	162

* Patients with mixed clinical pictures are included under each relevant heading.

disorder'. These patients have diminution or loss of two or more reflexes with proximal weakness and wasting. As well as being the most frequent type of disorder this is also the one which is most likely to be missed as these patients are often severely ill with carcinoma and confined to bed and any muscular weakness may well be attributed to the nonspecific effects of cachexia.

In addition to the 1465 patients seen other patients were specially referred to us because of symptoms of carcinomatous neuromyopathy, and we have given the incidence in these two groups separately. As might be expected there was a considerable difference between them as the neuromuscular syndromes are more easily missed than are the florid pictures. Exact classification of patients with carcinomatous neuromyopathy is often difficult because in any patient more than one part of the nervous system may be affected. Patients with mixed clinical pictures are included under each relevant heading in Table 17.

This tendency to involvement of more than one part of the nervous system is characteristic of the carcinomatous neuromyopathies. The neurological symptoms may develop either before, at the same time as or after those of the neoplasm. If the symptoms of the neuromyopathy develop before those of the cancer, it is reasonable to suppose that the cancer was present from the onset of neurological symptoms but so small as to be undetectable by usual diagnostic methods. This illustrates well that the extent and severity of the neuromyopathy is independent of the size of the neoplasm.

THE ENCEPHALOPATHIES

Dr Dayan and Dr Corsellis have described multifocal leucoencephalopathy and the acute encephalitides associated with malignancy. There is, however, one other type of encephalopathy which presents a very striking clinical picture.

Subacute cerebellar degeneration
This is a relatively uncommon form of carcinomatous neuromyopathy (Brain & Wilkinson 1965). Over the course of a few weeks or occasionally days the patient develops severe bilateral disturbances of cerebellar function producing inability to stand, gross ataxia of the arms and severe dysarthria so that the speech may become unintelligible. There may also be mental disturbances. In severe cases the patient may be so disabled that he cannot sit up in bed. The primary growth is most

frequently a bronchial carcinoma, and it is of interest that carcinoma of the ovary is the next most common neoplasm. The CSF often shows changes including pleocytosis, and a rise of protein with a paretic Lange.

The wide variety of symptoms and signs found in the encephalitis groups is the result of the differing distribution and severity of lesions in the nervous system. The duration of the neurological illness as a whole varies considerably, and in this series was from 5 to 20 months. In some cases the symptoms cease to progress and the patient remains in an unchanged neurological state for months or even years: in one case for six years. Patients with severe involvement of bulbar or spinal motor neurones may show a progressive course until death in a few weeks.

THE MYELOPATHIES

The spinal cord is involved in several types of carcinomatous neuro-myopathy and may be the primary site of damage to the nervous system. Alternatively cord changes may be found in association with encephalomyelitis and subacute cerebellar degeneration.

Motor neurone disease

One of the more distinct clinical pictures is that of the motor neurone type of carcinomatous neuromyopathy. In this the neurological disorder closely resembles motor neurone disease and occurs in association with various types of growth (Brain, Croft & Wilkinson 1965). The clinical features are similar to those of classic motor neurone disease having a combination of upper and lower motor neurone symptoms and signs though on the whole the disease tends to run a rather more benign course than does classical motor neurone disease. As in other types of neuromyopathy the symptoms and signs of the neurological disorder may precede the finding of the neoplasm.

Subacute necrotic myelopathy

This is a rare form of myelopathy associated with malignant disease in which there is massive necrosis in the cord (Mancall & Rosales 1964). In this condition the patient develops subacutely an ascending sensorimotor myelopathy which usually does not extend above the dorsal cord though occasionally the cervical region is involved. The paraplegia is generally flaccid with loss of reflexes: death may occur within two months. Findings in the CSF are variable but there is often an increase in cells or protein possibly associated with a paretic Lange. In other cases the fluid is normal.

Sensory neuropathy (ganglioradiculitis)
This is one of the less common of the carcinomatous neuropathies but the clinical syndrome is a dramatic one. The clinical course is subacute and the disability reaches its maximum in a few months and thereafter remains unchanged, though in the final stage of the illness the patient may develop moderate muscular weakness and mental disturbance. In one of our patients the severe sensory neuropathy developed overnight and remained virtually unchanged after that for many months until the patient died (Croft, Henson, Urich & Wilkinson 1965). The clinical disability is severe but not always symmetrical. In the early stages there may be backache and the patient may have distressing paraesthesiae in the limbs. Extensive sensory loss occurs affecting all forms of sensation both superficial and deep. At first the loss may be of segmental distribution but later tends to become universal affecting all the limbs and the trunk though not necessarily symmetrically. The main disability is the gross sensory ataxia which more or less cripples the patient. Power is normal although the patient has difficulty in using his muscles because of the virtual deafferentation of the limbs. The tendon reflexes are lost. The CSF protein tends to be raised in the active stages with levels as high as 200 mg/100 ml. In this type of neuropathy the neurological symptoms often occur well before any symptoms of neoplasm are present and sometimes the underlying carcinoma is only found at autopsy though its presence may have been suspected for many months. The interval between the onset of neurological symptoms and death of the patient has varied between six months and two years. The underlying neoplasm was a bronchial carcinoma of the oat cell type in three-quarters of the cases, and there was a high proportion of women. It was of interest that of the patients in whom specific antibrain antibodies in sera and cerebrospinal fluid were found by Wilkinson (1964) all but one had a sensory neuropathy.

Peripheral sensorimotor neuropathy
This type of mixed neuropathy is much more common than pure sensory neuropathy. Of 162 patients with carcinomatous neuromyo-

pathy peripheral sensory neuropathy was found in 36 (22 %). In a recent study (Croft, Urich & Wilkinson 1967) it was found possible to divide the patients into three groups. Firstly, patients known to have a carcinoma who may develop mild symptoms of peripheral neuropathy in the terminal stages of their illness. In such cases the neuropathy does not add greatly to the patient's disability. Secondly, those in whom the peripheral neuropathy is a severe disorder of subacute, and occasionally acute onset the patients often presenting with neurological syndromes. In the third type, which is similar to the second, the neuropathy follows a remitting and sometimes relapsing course. As with other types of carcinomatous neuromyopathy the clinical pictures tend to be mixed and peripheral sensorimotor neuropathy may occur in association with other forms. Carcinoma of the lung is again the most common primary neoplasm and accounts for about 50% of patients. Other responsible growths include carcinoma of the breast, stomach, colon, pancreas, body of the uterus and cervix, together with such disorders as Hodgkin's disease, malignant lymphoma and reticulum cell sarcoma of the pelvis. In the remitting and relapsing group, in which there were eight patients, the peripheral neuropathy showed a conspicuous clinical improvement and in some cases one or more subsequent relapses. The CSF protein may be considerably raised, the highest level found being 360 mg/100 l. There was a tendency for the protein to be higher in the acute stages of the disease and to fall when the condition became quiescent or improved. The cell count was rarely significantly raised but sometimes the Lange was paretic though this did not necessarily coincide with the high CSF protein level.

The striking difference in the natural history of the irreversible sensory neuropathy and the occasionally remitting peripheral sensorimotor neuropathy is presumably related to the site of the lesion. When severe neuronal loss occurs as in ganglioradiculitis it is improbable that any significant improvement can occur. Where the disorder is in part due to segmental demyelination of the peripheral nerve the possibilities of recovery are much greater.

CONCLUSIONS

While many of the syndromes produced remotely by malignant disease are now well recognized their pathogenesis remains obscure. It is necessary to explain, among other things, the variable time relationship between the growth and the neurological damage, the independence of the size of the primary growth, and the fact that only about 6% of patients with malignant disease develop these interesting syndromes. It is not necessary to postulate that all of the diverse remote effects produced by carcinoma are the results of a single pathological process. Some may be found to be the result of a specific virus infection while others may have a purely hormonal basis. On the other hand, it may be that in cases where a virus is incriminated the neurological disturbance results from an abnormal response to a commonly occurring virus, the altered response being caused by some polypeptide secreted by the primary tumour.

REFERENCES

AUCHÉ M. (1890) Des névrites périphériques chez les cancéreux. *Rév. Med. (Paris)*, **10**, 785–807.

BRAIN (LORD) & ADAMS R.D. (1965) In: *The Remote Effects of Cancer on the Nervous System*, Lord Brain and F.H.Norris (eds). New York, p. 216.

BRAIN (LORD), CROFT P.B. & WILKINSON M. (1965) Motor neurone disease as a manifestation of neoplasm. *Brain*, **88**, 479–500.

BRAIN W.R., DANIEL P.M. & GREENFIELD J.G. (1951) Subacute cortical cerebellar degeneration and its relation to carcinoma. *J. Neurol. Neurosurg. Psychiat.* **14**, 59–75.

BRAIN (LORD) & WILKINSON M. (1965) Subacute cerebellar degeneration associated with neoplasms. *Brain*, **88**, 465–478.

CROFT P.B., HENSON R.A., URICH H. & WILKINSON P.C. (1965) Sensory neuropathy with bronchial carcinoma. *Brain*, **88**, 501–514.

CROFT P.B., URICH H. & WILKINSON M. (1967) Peripheral neuropathy of sensori-motor type and malignant disease. *Brain*, **90**, 31–66.

CROFT P.B. & WILKINSON M. (1965) Incidence of carcinomatous neuromyopathy with various types of carcinoma. *Brain*, **88**, 427–434.

DENNY-BROWN D. (1948) Primary sensory neuropathy with muscular changes associated with carcinoma. *J. Neurol. Neurosurg. Psychiat.* **11**, 73–87.

LENNOX B. & PRITCHARD S. (1950) Association of bronchial carcinoma and peripheral neuritis. *Quart. J. Med.* **19**, 97–109.

MANCALL E.L. & ROSALES R.K. (1964) Necrotising myelopathy associated with visceral carcinoma. *Brain*, **87**, 639–656.

WILKINSON P.C. (1964) Serological findings in carcinomatous neuropathy. *Lancet*, i, 1301–1303.

The Pathology of Carcinomatous
Neurological Syndromes

H. Urich

Inflammatory lesions similar to those described by Corsellis in the cerebral hemispheres occur in the lower parts of the neuraxis, particularly the brain stem and the spinal cord (Henson, Russell & Wilkinson 1954, Henson, Hoffman & Urich 1965). In the brain stem neuronal destruction, focal or diffuse microglial activation and perivascular lymphocytic infiltration is seen predominantly in the medulla where it tends to involve the inferior olives, the floor of the fourth ventricle and a variety of motor and sensory nuclei ('bulbar encephalitis', Fig. 56). The process may extend in continuity into the spinal cord, which may also be involved independently ('myelitis', Fig. 57). The brunt of the damage falls on the anterior horns, but the posterior horns and

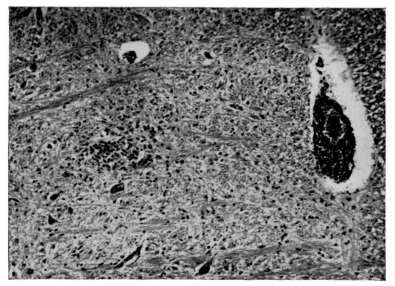

FIGURE 56. Case B/62 Bulbar encephalitis: heavy lymphocytic cuffing and microglial nodule in medulla. Haematoxylin and eosin. × 140.

Clarke's columns may also be affected. The lesions are usually most severe in the cervical segments, but may be scattered throughout the length of the cord.

A similar process affecting the posterior root ganglia ('ganglioradiculitis', Fig. 58) forms the anatomical substrate of sensory neuropathy (Denny-Brown 1948, Croft, Henson, Urich & Wilkinson 1965). Patchy

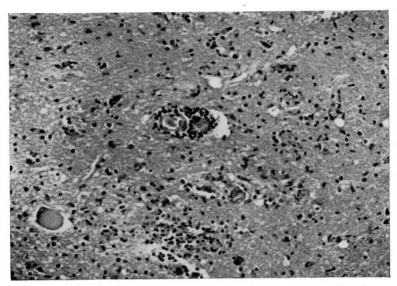

FIGURE 57. Case B/69 Myelitis: loss of nerve cells, microglial proliferation and sparse perivascular cuffing in anterior horn of cervical cord. Haematoxylin and eosin. × 180.

lymphocytic infiltration accompanies severe destruction of ganglion cells with phagocytosis and ultimate formation of residual nodules of pyknotic capsule cells. The efferent fibres of the ganglia in the posterior roots and columns undergo degeneration. The damage is usually widespread, but individual ganglia and their fibres may escape.

Sensory neuropathy is often associated with a minor degree of encephalomyelitis and, conversely, minimal ganglioradiculitis is often found in cases presenting as bulbar encephalitis or myelitis.

The pathology of syndromes affecting predominantly the motor system ('motor neurone disease', Brain, Croft & Wilkinson 1965) has not been worked out satisfactorily. Only in one case were typical lesions of amyotrophic lateral sclerosis present and in view of their association with tumours of doubtful malignancy (pulmonary 'tumour-lets') the combination may well be coincidental. Another case, associated with a long-standing carcinoma of the breast, showed almost total loss of anterior horn cells throughout the spinal cord (Fig. 59) but no other lesions. The remaining two cases showed minimal, barely

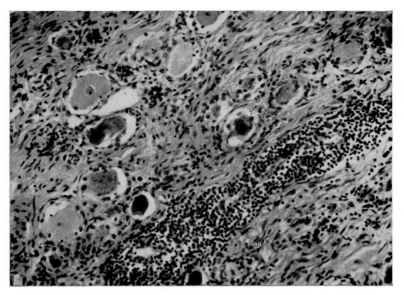

FIGURE 58. Case B/62 Ganglioradiculitis: lymphocytic infiltration, degeneration of nerve cells and nodules of Nageotte in posterior root ganglion C6. Haematoxylin and eosin. × 170.

perceptible, loss of anterior horn cells, mild destructive lesions in posterior root ganglia and posterior columns and, in one instance only, degeneration of the cortico-spinal tracts.

The mixed sensorimotor neuropathy is due to lesions in the peripheral nerves where both demyelination with preservation of axons and axonal destruction may be present in variable proportions (Lennox & Pritchard 1950, Croft, Urich & Wilkinson 1967). Sparse lymphocytic infiltration may be found in some cases (Fig. 60). The spinal nerve roots may be similarly affected. In the rare instances of severe destruction of the posterior roots degenerative changes may be found in the posterior root ganglia and the posterior columns of the spinal cord.

In the well-known cerebellar degenerations (Brain, Daniel & Green-field 1951, Brain & Wilkinson 1965) the main lesion is severe, often subtotal loss of Purkinje cells with preservation of other layers of the cerebellar cortex (Fig. 61). This is usually an isolated finding, but in rare instances it may be accompanied by degeneration of the long tracts or associated with other types of carcinomatous neuropathy.

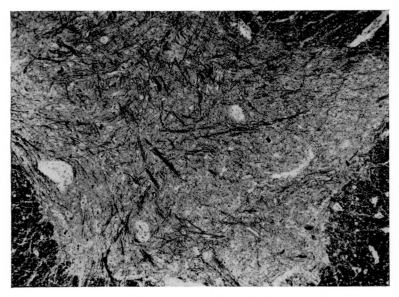

FIGURE 59. Case B/78 'Motor neurone disease': almost total loss of large neurones in anterior horn of segment L5. Klüver and Barrera's method. × 45.

The author has no experience of the rare necrotizing myelopathy associated with carcinoma (Mancall & Rosales 1964).

In evaluating the pathogenetic implications of these findings it is important to emphasize that any of these lesions may occur, albeit rarely, in the absence of malignant neoplasms. They appear to form a heterogeneous group of disorders and it is difficult to uphold the view that they are all due to a similar pathogenetic mechanism. It is probably justifiable to consider the inflammatory and the degenerative syndromes separately, although the separation may be difficult on morphological grounds alone. On one hand cases do occur in which both types of

lesion are found side by side, on the other it must be admitted that the
end result of a burnt-out inflammatory process or of one in which
the cellular reaction has been suppressed by treatment may be indistinguishable from a purely degenerative condition. Yet the curious
association of encephalomyelitis and ganglioradiculitis with oat cell
carcinoma of the bronchus in contrast with the wide range of neoplasms

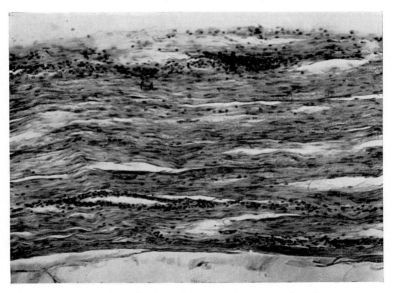

FIGURE 60. Case B/54 Peripheral Neuropathy: sparse lymphocytic infiltration in ulnar nerve. Van Gieson. × 150.

which may accompany degenerative neuropathies sets the inflammatory
group apart. This group clinically covers a wide range of syndromes
from memory defects to sensory neuropathy, but pathologically is
fairly homogeneous both in its relation to the type of primary tumour,
in its pattern of cellular reaction and in the co-existence of lesions in
the various regions commonly affected.

The striking feature of the cellular reaction is its resemblance to that
seen in the common types of virus infections of the central nervous
system. It is, however, essential to avoid the fallacious identification
of inflammation with infection. The presence of inflammation indicates
a type of host reaction and throws little light on aetiological factors.

16

In the examples illustrated here the main features are the accumulation of immunologically competent cells in perivascular spaces and mobilization and activation of macrophages. These represent an immune reaction which may be directed against a variety of antigens, both exogenous and endogenous. The viral theory has recently received support from Walton, Tomlinson & Pearce (1968) who found structures

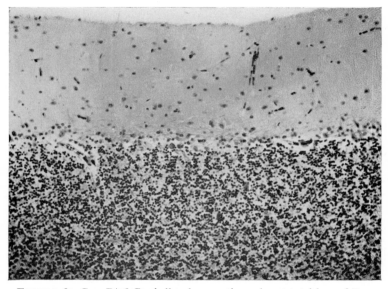

FIGURE 61. Case B/46 Cerebellar degeneration: almost total loss of Purkinje cells in cerebellar cortex. Klüver-Barrera. × 130.

resembling virus particles in electron micrographs of the spinal cord in a case of subacute myelitis associated with Hodgkin's disease. On the other hand Wilkinson (1964) found circulating auto-antibodies to a component of neuronal cytoplasm in cases of sensory neuropathy. It is tempting to suggest that these antibodies are directed against common antigenic determinants shared by tumour cells and neurones but these have never been demonstrated. It is equally possible that the immune response is provoked by an infective agent sharing antigens with nerve cells.

The possible role of viruses in the degenerative conditions is even more open to doubt. Little is known of the role of infective agents in the production of peripheral neuropathies, but here again an immune response of delayed hypersensitivity type may be invoked.

Little thought was given in the past to the possibility that selective destruction of certain cell types and of systems of fibre tracts without any evidence of host reaction could be due to infective agents. Recent discoveries of the effects of slow viruses on the central nervous system offer a new, and possibly fruitful, field of investigation in this obscure branch of cerebral pathology.

REFERENCES

BRAIN (LORD), CROFT P.B. & WILKINSON M. (1965) Motorneurone disease as a manifestation of neoplasm. *Brain*, **88**, 479–499.

BRAIN W.R., DANIEL P.M. & GREENFIELD J.G. (1951) Subacute cortical cerebellar degeneration and its relation to carcinoma. *J. Neurol. Neurosurg. Psychiat.* **14**, 59–75.

BRAIN (LORD) & WILKINSON M. (1965) Subacute cerebellar degenerations associated with neoplasms. *Brain*, **88**, 465–479.

CROFT P.B., HENSON R.A., URICH H. & WILKINSON P.C. (1965) Sensory neuropathy with bronchial carcinoma. *Brain*, **88**, 501–514.

CROFT P.B., URICH H. & WILKINSON M. (1967) Peripheral neuropathy of sensorimotor type and malignant disease. *Brain*, **90**, 31–66.

DENNY-BROWN D. (1948) Primary sensory neuropathy with muscular change associated with carcinoma. *J. Neurol. Neurosurg. Psychiat.* **11**, 73–87.

HENSON R.A., HOFFMAN H.L. & URICH H. (1965) Encephalomyelitis with carcinoma. *Brain*, **88**, 449–464.

HENSON R.A., RUSSELL D.S. & WILKINSON M. (1954) Carcinomatous neuropathy and myopathy: a clinical and pathological study. *Brain*, **77**, 82–120.

LENNOX B. & PRITCHARD S. (1950) Association of bronchial carcinoma and peripheral neuritis. *Quart. J. Med.* **19**, 97–109.

MANCALL E.L. & ROSALES R.K. (1964) Necrotising myelopathy associated with visceral carcinoma. *Brain*, **87**, 639–656.

WALTON J.N., TOMLINSON B.E. & PEARCE G.W. (1968) Subacute 'poliomyelitis' and Hodgkins disease. *J. neurol. Sci.* **6**, 435–445.

WILKINSON P.C. (1964) Serological findings in carcinomatous neuropathy. *Lancet*, i, 1301–1303.

Discussion on Viruses and Malignant Disease of the Nervous System

CHAIRMAN: MacCALLUM: I thought it might be helpful if we sought for some comment from disinterested parties, so we have asked Dr Offord if he would like to say something from the viewpoint of molecular biology. We have been fortunate to have Professor Calvin here and he may also like to comment. Then, before our concluding general discussion, Dr Spillane will give a clinician's reaction to what we have heard.

OFFORD: About 50% of my knowledge of animal viruses has been acquired this morning. However, I hope that an examination of the difficulties of this subject by one who is occasionally called a 'molecular biologist' may be of some interest and help to bring out the points I feel the organizers of this conference wish me to make.

First, why should viruses *not* cause malignancy? They so clearly interfere with those very processes and mechanisms which are essential to the maintenance of the integrity of a cell or mass of cells, that it is difficult to see how the possibility could be questioned. We have been given a list of animal viruses implicated in this way but the phenomenon is not restricted to this class. For instance, a whole range of plant viruses, the so-called 'witches' broom' viruses, cause grave disturbance in cell differentiation in the host. They may, for instance, cause an aerial potato tuber to be formed from the stem or leaf tissue, or cause the proliferation of what are morphologically root hairs at perhaps the crown of the plant.

Viruses, then, may be expected to have the ability to cause malignancy, and have in several instances been shown to do so: though they do not always. Why do cell biologists look at cell transformation brought about by viruses rather than by other simpler agents? Viruses, considered as chemicals, are so complex that their use may need justification. One of the most powerful tools of molecular biology is to bring about, and select for, genetic variations that throw light on the mechanism under study. This is particularly appropriate for transformation, which is brought about by some

231

aspect of the behaviour of a gene. To use this approach in chemical transformation one would have to modify the cell genes, of which there are, to say the least, a very large number. In the case of virus transformation a viral gene is quite clearly involved and since there are usually less than ten of them, the problem of applying the method is simplified by several orders of magnitude.

A subsidiary question is why a virus like SV40, which in nature is exclusively a pathogen to primates, with no recorded association with malignancy, should be used to study transformation and largely in the cells of newborn rodents; and how applicable the results are to man? I do not work in this field but I suppose it is a question of experimental convenience; and that reliance is placed, doubtless well justified, on the essential similarity of vital processes across the species.

I would like now to say a little more of the actual process of transformation, how it works and why it should work, and then go on to examine the bearing this may have on what I regard as the allied problem of latency in virus infections.

One of the major features of malignancy is loss by the cell of the ability to recognize 'stop' signals, this being associated with antigenic changes on the surface of that cell. Transformation of cells in culture provides a convincing *in vitro* model of just this process. Here again, from the nature of viruses, one might expect this to happen. It has been known since Beijerinck discovered viruses in the 1890's that they are almost exclusively associated with growing tissue. Thus, particularly in the case of animals, for a virus to prosper some mechanism for bringing about the unrestrained growth of the cells which it infects would be desirable: and this is a characteristic of malignant cells. If the virus does do this, it seems to act by affecting the surface properties of the cell membrane. This is also of interest since animal viruses are frequently produced at membranes, and therefore some change at the membrane, particularly some slight degeneration or weakening of the membrane structure, would be useful to the virus. As an interpolation here, I was interested that the Rous sarcoma virus requires 'helpers'. It is not impossible that these helper viruses are doing just this particular job for it. Alternatively the situation may be analogous to that of another plant virus, Tobacco Rattle Virus. Here, it seems that the original gene has split into two parts and now resides in two particles of distinct though closely related morphology. One gene, and thus one type of particle, is able to bring about the symptoms of infection, but the other, entirely without effect when alone, is needed in addition to bring about the assembly of finished particles and attain the maximum rate of multiplication of the combined pathogen.

The effect of viruses on the surface properties of the cell in transformation may therefore be seen as an example of natural economy in which some process normally used for other things, may, under the right circumstances, give rise to a pathogenic phenomenon. Similarly, transforming virus has an effect on cell metabolism, and here too mechanisms used in virus multiplication also seem suitable for use in the transformation process. Thus one of the earliest phenomena noted when cells in tissue culture are infected by virus is the activation of often previously dormant synthetic reactions in the cell. Suddenly, there is a tremendous burst of synthesis, both of protein and nucleic acid. It is important to note that this occurs at a point before it is clear whether the cell is to die or just to be transformed and become 'malignant'. Here again this is the sort of thing a virus might be expected to do. It must stimulate cell metabolism if it itself is to be synthesized; it must reactivate the machinery which is normally used for replicating cellular DNA in order to bring about the replication of its own DNA and protein and thus multiply itself.

It is of great interest that in this burst of metabolic activity virtually the first thing that follows the introduction of virus is the production of the 'T' antigen, mentioned earlier. This protein, not detectable before, appears in the cell nucleus and its precise nature appears to depend on the species of virus involved and not on the species of cell. It has been suggested that it is some sort of activating molecule and over-rides the normal mechanism regulating gene expression and providing for a proper balance in the relative amounts of the constituents of the cell. Elucidation of the exact nature and function of the T antigen is thus awaited with great interest.

These and allied observations reinforce the impression that viruses play an important part in transformation at several of its stages. Does this help us to understand the clinical problem of malignant disease? One important question is when does the direct action of the virus cease? Does transformation of a single cell simply cause its unrestrained proliferation and thus produce a persisting effect of malignancy, without further participation of virus? Alternatively, does the virus or part of it remain in the cell, undergoing replication with it all the way down the life history of the transformed cell line? The answers are beginning to be known. It seems clear, to take SV40 as an example, that virus particles or components thereof are not to be found in transformed cell progeny by any present physical or biochemical technique. However, by administering certain biological stimuli to the cell culture, some cell generations later than the original transformation, a crop of perfectly normal SV40 particles are obtained. (I will discuss the nature of the stimulus later.) This implies that the viral DNA lies hidden in the transformed cell progeny, with the function of producing progeny particles lying dormant. Thus, one need not expect to see virus particles on electron microscopy, since one can usually see only the protein part which may not be made. However, we cannot assume that the essential part of the virus, the genetic strand of DNA or RNA, is not there.

We have now approached the problem of latency, one of the overall subjects of this Symposium. We have seen a virus lying latent and not, in the normal sense of the word, detectable, until a biological event occurs which enables it to appear and multiply. In some cases this latency appears to involve a disturbance of metabolism which emerges as 'malignancy'. It is, however, reasonable to speculate that the disappearance of the virus without producing immediate malignant symptoms, involves the same type of mechanism. The two have sufficient in common to make the idea worth further consideration. (It must not be forgotten, however, that a single virus particle would be very hard to detect, yet might be present and thus latent in a different sense.)

As a basis for what follows, I would like to make a brief mention of the molecular processes which are thought to transmit the hereditable information in cell and virus replication. It is now held, with almost theological rigour, that the chemical structure of DNA, or, in the case of some viruses, RNA, is the ultimate seat of hereditable information. This chemical structure is able to influence the structure of nucleic acids synthesized in its presence, by a hydrogen bonding process, to such an extent that the DNA molecule acts as a template for its own reproduction. This reproduction can be of progeny DNA, which is destined to provide the same service for the next generation, or progeny RNA which provides for the needs of the present generation. This RNA (the 'messenger') carries the imprint of the DNA to sites of protein synthesis mainly in the cytoplasm, where its structure influences the structure of the proteins synthesized. The direction of the RNA synthesis is known as transcription; the direction of protein synthesis is called translation. Infection by a virus can now be seen as the arrival of an extraneous DNA or RNA which seizes the transcription and translation process of the cell and turns it to the production of components peculiar to itself. This type of acute infection cycle is called 'productive'. Infection leading to transformation or latency is not so simple. The DNA arrives and must be able to transcribe itself, since, as the extent of subsequent stimulated virus recovery shows, it can keep pace with cell division and lie dormant in nearly every cell. It may even become incorporated structurally into the host's DNA. Since whole virus is not normally seen, either the transcription to messenger RNA or the translation to virus protein must be suppressed. It is on the nature and means of this suppression that the discussion of the mechanism of this type of latency turns.

At present no overwhelming evidence supports either site for suppression. However, some rather interesting observations favour suppression of the *translation* process. In particular, analytical tests on the cytoplasm of transformed cells show the presence of virus specific messenger RNA. It is not possible to say whether or not the total expected amount of messenger is present, but at least part of the transcription process is operating. If translation is at fault, can one see how this could occur? I would like, in closing, to mention one possible mechanism, not because I or its originators regard it as proven, but because it illustrates very well one type of approach to the problem.

Messenger RNA influences protein structure by the use of what are called coding triplets. Early in the evolution of living matter, some arbitrary relationships were established between nucleic acid structure and the protein structure determined by it. This involved the nucleotide sequence of the former, and the amino-acid sequence of the latter. Since there are four different types of nucleotide, there are 64 different 'words' which can be made by combining them three at a time. It has been found that in nearly all cases whenever a given triplet occurs in the nucleic acid sequence a particular amino acid follows in the protein sequence. Since there are only 20 amino acids to be coded for in this way, some amino acids must be specified by more than one triplet. The suggestion is that of the possible range of triplets calling forth a given amino acid one is only used very rarely. As a result the machinery which translates triplets into amino acids might lose the ability to 'recognize' this rarely used triplet. If the virus uses the triplet and the host cell does not, the proteins relying on that triplet for their completion will not appear, since at that stage the DNA could only switch to the more common triplet by the highly improbable event of a favourable chance mutation. This idea becomes particularly interesting because the biological stimulus for virus recovery which I mentioned previously is the fusion of the cytoplasm of a transformed cell with that of another type. If the second cell has the missing part of the machinery, virus multiplication will resume.

I hope this survey will serve to illustrate the approaches to your problems which are possible for the type of biologist I have been asked to represent.

One final point, I was most interested to see the photographs of virus particles in whole tissue extracts. Knowing the difficulties of seeing particles in such murky material, I wondered if routine purification of the appropriate fraction of material from other pathological conditions might be rewarding. Purification might, of course, destroy some viruses, but it would allow those not destroyed to be seen more readily: and some conditions, not at present recognized as virus associated, might well show up particles.

CALVIN: I wasn't really aware that I would be called upon to speak this morning. When I was told about this meeting, I really came to listen rather than to speak. However, now that I have been called up, I would like to present an idea and then ask a question, though not in regard to the things that Dr Offord has described. These latter seem to me a very reasonable and rational way of having the same condition appear sometimes in the genome and sometimes not, which is the kind of thing which has been repeatedly described in the symposium in the last two days. I came particularly interested in yesterday's discussion which Dr Offord didn't refer to directly. This is the question of the physical-chemical nature of the infective agent in Scrapie and Kuru. In view of the fact that Dr Offord did not address himself to this, may I say just a word or two about it. I must say that I hadn't until yesterday afternoon seen as much of the physics and chemistry of the presumed agent which transmits the disease by experimental methods as I saw yesterday, and in view of that I would like to suggest that there are alternatives, or at least it is possible to reconcile the existing dogma which you have heard here briefly described, with both the points of view that were presented yesterday and with the physics and chemistry that was determined on the experimental form of the infective or transmitting agent.

As you have seen, it can sometimes be part of the genome and sometimes not, and in that sense I think it is quite conceivable that the two conflicting points of view that we heard yesterday can be reconciled, although I don't really want to go into the details of that right now. I would rather refer to the suggestion of the actual structure of the agent that might be deducible from the evidence presented yesterday on the actual physical-chemical entity that is involved. I think that Dr Hunter's suggestion that it might be associated with a piece of the cell membrane is certainly an acceptable one. In fact, as I listened to his talk this is the kind of structure which arose in my mind. I did not think of it at that time as a piece of the cell membrane because I was thinking as a physical and organic chemist so I thought in terms of the molecules that one would have to assemble to produce the result he described. He has described it as a piece of membrane, but the assembly of molecules that came to my mind was precisely the assembly that we are now currently exploring as possible means of constructing a cell membrane. Now without enumerating all of the physics and chemistry which he put on the blackboard yesterday, I will try, if I can, to remember the essential pieces.

First of all, the two most important were the resistance of the agent to heat and to ultraviolet light and this has caused some consternation amongst the biologists and even the molecular biologists, although I think it doesn't really have to. On the other hand, he also presented for the first time, at least to my eyes, a series of conditions to which the agent was labile and these conditions were 6 M salt, 6 M urea, 80°C after a fluorocarbon, and 90% phenol. I don't recall whether there were any others but those are the ones I got. All of these, together with the two resistance conditions, ultraviolet light and heat, can be accounted for in terms of the physical-chemical structure which is derived in much the same way that Dr Hunter suggested; as an invagination of a cell membrane which is then pinched off as a separate entity and the result of those conditions in that entity will be membranous in character, that is, it will have the same kind of character as the cell membrane itself. Now in order to fulfil the requirements as they have so far been described, this would have to be a lipid which has negative charges on the outside and in the centre would be the nucleic acid which accounts for its replicability. The lipid outside structure would have to be very special in its character. It would have to have multiple unsaturation, a large number of double bonds, as well as a number of vicinal dihydroxy groups, to represent, first, protection against ultraviolet and, secondly, the susceptibility to periodate. Both of these are quite common chemically and the presence of this kind of structure, or this kind of unit, in the outside wall of the infective particle would indeed produce the kind of results that Dr Hunter described.

Then, in conclusion, I would like to ask a question which perhaps either the genetic school or the experimental school could answer, and that is: when the animal is infected by injection, whatever route the injection is achieved, does this infectivity eventually find its way into the genome and then can it be transmitted by the reproductive action of the animal?

CHAIRMAN: Thank you, Dr Calvin. Your question will be answered later but we must now turn to our final discussion.

SPILLANE: I think one would have to be harbouring a very powerful antibody to imagination if one was not to profit from this meeting. What a catalytic agent the virus is. The people who have been drawn into this discussion seem to be almost everyone. Professor Darlington reminded us that a virus may have a history as complex as its host. We know some of them are ancient, those of smallpox, and polio-myelitis, but new ones can descend on us from the primates and other animals, as has recently happened in Germany. The dual potentiality of the provirus seems to make the clinician's distinction of infection and heredity much less fundamental after all. The neurologist of 1968 can see major contributions in the clinical field not only of techniques but of ideas, stemming from virology. Since 1898 when Loeffler demonstrated a filter passing particle in foot and mouth disease, development has been extraordinary. The passage of St. Louis virus encephalitis from man to animals by Muckenfuss in 1933, a wide range of work on the polio virus, and the recognition of innumer-able neurotropic viruses and their clinical pictures has culminated in this recent concept of the slow and latent virus—perhaps the most important contribution of all. If this provides a possible clue to the causes of chronic degenerative neurological disease the clinical neurolo-gist will indeed be grateful. It is an old observation that motor neurone disease occurs in people who have had poliomyelitis in childhood.

We know that Parkinsonism indistinguishable from degenerative paralysis agitans follows a virus infection. In clinical neurology we must search for cures and perhaps the slow virus concept and the ultimate end of this research will provide these. I suppose the significance of any symposium is not so much what is said as where it leads: and by this criterion ours should be very worthwhile.

General Discussion

Chairman
F. O. MacCallum

MacCallum: Thank you, Dr Spillane. Who would, like to start off the general discussion?

Almeida: I think that there has been a great deal of discussion in this symposium about the presence and possible importance of antigen/antibody aggregates in brain tissue. Whether or not such aggregates do exist should be capable of elucidation by use of electron microscope techniques. Fernando & Movat (*Amer. J. Path.* **43**, 381, 1963) showed that it is possible to visualize antigen/antibody aggregates in thin sections using ferritin as a label. A variation of this technique could be employed whereby ferritin-labelled antiglobulin antibody could be reacted with the brain tissue in question. The resulting thin sections would then be examined for the presence of ferritin molecules which should be localized in the vicinity of antigen/antibody complexes. This approach would have the additional advantage that it would not be necessary to know the nature of the antigen implicated.

Tyrrell: I would like to make a comment on a slightly related subject, arising from Professor Urich's talk. There is a tendency to say that either there is an auto-immune process or there is a virus infection and this may be a false antithesis. A recent example which appears to be proving this point is that New Zealand black mice, which are known to develop an auto-immune disease and which show Coombs positive tests on the red blood cells, in fact, appear to develop this disease because they are infected with a virus which is very difficult to transmit, but can be transmitted and which can be demonstrated by electronmicroscopy. So sometimes it may be that the auto-immune process has been initiated because of the virus infection and just because you find one or the other it does not mean to say that the other half of the process will not be active as well.

241

TOMLINSON: I would like to put a question to the Hammersmith team about interpretation of electronmicrographs. Classically, viruses have been looked for as transmissible infectious agents, but increasingly we find them being looked for under the electronmicroscope. Professor Waterson talked of the PML 'virus' which has not yet been transmitted. There has been a good deal of confusion caused over various blobs found in electronmicrographs from leukaemic material. Would either of them care to comment on what criteria should be employed now and in the future to decide whether things seen in electronmicrographs really are viruses or not, so that as new agents are looked for people do not get led on wrong trails?

ALMEIDA: I think we could take this in conjunction with a question from Dr Hughes yesterday, when he showed his thin section pictures that looked like herpes type, but he was not completely convinced as to whether they were or not.

Results gained from the electron microscope are strictly non-biological in type. Particles seen in the electron microscope are in the real meaning of the word artefacts. Because of this it becomes very important to look at suspected virus particles with more than one technique. Many viruses with thin sectioning appear as little round blobs but the same particles with negative staining reveal geometrically arranged capsids that can be identified without hesitation. This is one of the reasons why we have been very anxious to use the negative staining technique on SSPE tissue so that we could show, as we have done, that the filaments present in thin sections do indeed display the herring-bone pattern typical of measles virus helix.

I think the particles Dr Hughes showed yesterday were virus particles but his case would be considerably strengthened if he were able by negative staining to show the presence of a geometrically arranged capsid.

DAYAN: I would like to make two points. First of all trying to speak as a quasi-clinician, when thinking of virus diseases of the nervous system we have perhaps thought for too long of cells, neurones or glial cells, either being destroyed by a virus or not being affected at all. From what we have seen of the molecular biology of viruses ought we not to be considering also the cells with disordered or perverted metabolism behaving in an abnormal fashion but still functioning to some extent? There is some evidence for this in the example of subacute sclerosing panencephalitis. There are now a number of cases described in which a very abnormal pattern of ganglioside synthesis has occurred within the CNS and this appears to be due to the virus infection; one might perhaps consider this within a wider context of other diseases.

A question to Professor Dick. He mentioned yesterday the problem of the epidemiology of subacute sclerosing panencephalitis. He mentioned how rare it apparently is in Northern Ireland but, dealing with a population that is only slightly larger than yours in Northern Ireland I have seen three cases in one year, two of which were highly atypical, the third was just rather odd. How many of these diseases in fact are we missing because the mechanisms of identifying, and particularly for registering them officially, are very poor?

HUNTER: I am sure all the workers in the Scrapie field are very grateful to Professor Calvin for his very interesting suggestion although I am not completely convinced. One point to bear in mind is that the resistance of the Scrapie agent to ultraviolet irradiation appears to be absolute and it is difficult to imagine that the odd photon would not get through. So perhaps if the type of structure that Professor Calvin suggests, really exists one would have to make a further postulation that perhaps the Scrapie agent contains a very simple repeating nucleic acid sequence such that a few breaks would still leave the informational sequence complete and I think that this is a possibility.

But to turn to another point I would like to put to Professor Waterson or one of the virologists. It is commonly assumed by virologists and molecular biologists, and Dr Offord so assumed, that viral transformation is effected by the nucleic acid component of the virus. But there is quite a bit of evidence that this may not always be the case. There is Defendi's work which has shown that the transformation ability is much more resistant to irradiation than the transmissibility of the agent. More recently, a paper in the *Journal of Experimental Medicine*, I am afraid I forget the authors, showed that while the transmissible agent, mouse leukaemia virus, could be eliminated in a conventional manner by ultraviolet radiation, the transformation ability, in human bone marrow cells, was completely resistant to ultraviolet radiation under their conditions. Of course when you have got the transformation in bone marrow cells, if it is

17

affected by the protein component of the virus you still have to use the intact cell for transmissibility but one is approaching a little more closely to the Scrapie type of situation and I wonder if Professor Waterson, or one of the other virologists, has any comments on this?

WATERSON: About the question of transmissibility of the agent and the power to transform a cell, obviously the Rous sarcoma virus, certainly the defective types which were mentioned, is not transmissible but it is capable of transforming. However, that does not mean that it does so without its nucleic acid and the actual part of the virus genome. You may only have to destroy quite a small part of the nucleic acid to stop it being transmitted and yet leave a large part intact.

DICK: I think Dr Dayan is quite right. We have really no idea of how many cases of subacute sclerosing panencephalitis there are but all I was trying to say is that when I was in Northern Ireland, where the population was fairly static and where specimens from most of the patients with this particular condition would likely come to the Pathology Department in Belfast, there were groups of three cases in one year, then one case over a 10-year period: before that a little group of three cases. The thing that struck me very much was this grouping, like your three cases in one year. Now, are you going to see no more for seven or eight years?

May I now ask one question? I was wondering, is there anything remarkable in the γ-globulins of these patients with the various neurological syndromes associated with carcinoma. Does anybody know anything about this?

MACCALLUM: Dr Croft, can you throw any light on this?

CROFT: No I am afraid I can't. I was going to take up the point that Dr Tyrrell made. He said that the auto-immune and the infectious theory were not inconsistent. The point, of course, is that the only cases in which the antibodies were found by Peter Wilkinson were, in fact, those which on histological grounds showed inflammatory changes.

URICH: I would like to support Dr Dayan in his plea for more epidemiological studies and that applies to all conditions we are discussing here. We would like to know much more about the incidence of the various conditions, both the established virus infections and the hypothetical ones in various parts of the world because I think that, what is now called geographical pathology, certainly can add a lot of hints in the direction of what are exogenous and what are endogenous factors in the development of the disease and can link the exogenous factors with known existing factors in various parts of the world.

ALPERS: Could Professor Waterson tell me if he could distinguish between polyoma and SV40 under the electronmicroscope. Because if he cannot I suggest that this agent in PML is more likely to be SV40, which is after all a primate virus, than polyoma.

MacCALLUM: Dr Alpers, can you tell us whether there has been any more work on attempted transmission of amyotrophic lateral sclerosis in the USA.

ALPERS: There has been more work done but there have been no positive results at all on amyotrophic lateral sclerosis; neither with material from the familial United States cases, the sporadic cases nor the cases from Guam.

WATERSON: About PML and polyoma and SV40 viruses: all these three viruses are 450 Å in diameter and of indistinguishable structure in the electronmicroscope and I cannot stress the latter too strongly. Recently there was a rather misleading leader, if that's not a contradiction in terms, in the *Lancet* headed 'polyoma and something or other' which implied that the electron microscope findings in PML suggested that the particles seen were mouse polyoma virus. Now there is no evidence on this whatsoever, all we can say is that the particles seen are indistinguishable morphologically from mouse polyoma and there is also no evidence, of course, that they are SV40. In every case that we hear about, we make an enquiry about whether they had polio vaccine, but can I stress again there is no evidence that this is polyoma virus of mice.

HUGHES: I would like to ask two questions. The first is to Professor Dick who yesterday, in his talk on subacute sclerosing panencephalitis, suggested the possibility that γ-globulin was locally manufactured

17§

in the brain. I wonder if he would suggest how this could be effected? Would the lymphocytes and plasma cells that migrated into the CNS then proceed to manufacture this antibody or does he know a source of lymphoid tissue in the CNS unknown to me? The second question is to Dr Dayan. This morning he showed us very beautifully the giant binucleated astrocytes which first took our attention in PML, and he also said the oligodendrocytes were involved. A few weeks ago I was in Boston and I saw most of the cases that Aström, Mancall & Richardson originally described. The sections of a further case came in whilst I was there and this case was similar in all respects, except that it lacked these abnormal astrocytes. This is to me rather reassuring because from the nature of the disease I would suspect that the important cell that is attacked is the oligodendrocyte and not the astrocyte. I wondered if these cells, which we are describing as astrocytes could be abnormal cells of some other glial type?

EARL: I would like to ask two questions which are really directed at the virologists and one of them I think has been answered in part. I would like to know whether they know of half a dozen more or less specific situations which in an experimental set up will activate virus infections that may be latent. If one is looking for reasons for the appearance of diseases that appear to be due to latent virus infections one way of course in which they might appear would be by the operation of some factor which may be well known to virologists in their experiments and which we could look for in clinical situations. The second question was one that may show my ignorance but it was whether the virus in progressive multifocal leucoencephalopathy could be the sort of virus that Professor Darlington was talking about which is in fact acting in one way as a hereditary particle and causing the Hodgkin's disease and in another way acting as an infectious agent in the brain.

MacCALLUM: I think there was a question to you, Professor Dick, about the formation of antibody in the CNS which has been worrying me also.

DICK: I have no secret knowledge of any secret mechanism of antibody formation in CNS but I presume that this antibody is formed by cells of the lymphocytic series which have got in there and are wandering about there, and Cohen & Bannister you may recall have actually found that cells in CSF are capable of forming both IgM and IgG.

MacCALLUM: In answer to Dr Earl I think that almost any kind of injury may activate latent infection. There's sunlight, cold, 'stress', immunosuppressive drugs, adrenalin and allergic shock, or perhaps even another virus. The patient of Marshall in Glasgow, was hit on the head with a golf ball and in a few days herpes encephalitis developed, so I think that if the limits of the MRC ethics will allow you to stimulate your patients I think you might easily find some trigger mechanism. It may not be the same mechanism which is most effective in different patients.

DAYAN: I agree with Dr Hughes that it is difficult to identify cells in the normal CNS—it's even more difficult in pathological states—but I think that some of these giant cells are probably astrocytes because one can show a progression from normal astrocytes towards these enormous giant cells. Some of the ones that are not too abnormal do show the silver staining characteristic of astrocytes but I would not regard it as being completely cut and dried. Also in subacute sclerosing panencephalitis there are many pyronophilic cells in the CNS, around blood vessels and scattered loosely in the cortex which can look like plasma cells. I presume that γ-globulin comes from them but the fluorescent anti-γ-globulin pictures published by Belfast and American workers have not shown anything like the number of fluorescent cells one would have liked to have seen.

PALLIS: In relation to Dr Earl's question, it seems to me there are two situations in which this relationship between a form of trauma and sudden multiplication of virus is so common that it probably needs a specific explanation. One is the patient who has a division of the sensory root of the trigeminal nerve for trigeminal neuralgia and then develops herpes simplex in the denervation territory, this is probably seen in something like 10%, or perhaps even more, patients having retrogasserian neurectomies. The other is the patient with flare up of varicella/zoster in the dermatome affected by say a secondary tumour or Paget's disease or some vertebral disorder.

MacCALLUM: I would put the incidence of herpes in the denervation area as closer to 90%.

WEBB: May I just throw one spanner in the works about this continual differentiation between the astrocytes and the oligodendrocyte. It seems to me that we lay much too much stress on the difference between these two cells when it seems highly likely that in fact one is possibly a rather more mature example of the other. It seems that electron microscopically they are really identical and I would like some comments from the pathologists.

MACCALLUM: Is Dr Udall here? You are interested in toxicology. I wonder if you have any comments on toxic changes, or other comments with regard to this morning's subject of cancer and the degenerative disease in the CNS. Do you have any ideas about this at all, whether this might be a toxin?

There are two other people we haven't heard from. Dr Harriman, have you got any comments or questions that you would like to ask?

HARRIMAN: The question that has puzzled me and perhaps the virologists might be able to answer it, is what is the relationship between the intranuclear inclusion, which has varying staining capabilities and the virus? What part of the virus is being shown in the light microscope? Is it the whole virus or is it part of the virus and can we be helped in any way by its staining characteristics? Secondly, in subacute sclerosing panencephalitis we often find very few intranuclear inclusions indeed and we call it SSP, whereas in other instances which are perhaps similar in their course, there are very numerous intranuclear inclusions indeed and they are then called Dawson's inclusion body encephalitis. Thirdly what about those rare examples which are called cytomegalic inclusion body disease? This is a sort of problem that meets the light microscopist who has not got, unfortunately, access to electronmicroscopy.

MACCALLUM: Professor Waterson, would you or Dr Tyrrell like to answer briefly on the question of inclusion bodies.

WATERSON: Could I first answer another question which has not been completely answered yet? Dr Earl asked about the PML virus—could this be as well as the cause of the PML also the cause of the Hodgkin's disease or whatever it is? Well yes—I think this is a very attractive hypothesis and the answer is we simply do not know but please let us have the brain from your next patient with PML who dies.

MacCallum: I think that Dr Harriman is still waiting for an answer.

Tyrrell: I think we must be very cautious about making any generaliza-tion about inclusions because there are many different sorts of viruses and even one sort of virus may make more than one sort of inclusion. For example, I showed some pictures of adenoviruses and a variety of basophilic and eosinophilic inclusions can occur inside the nucleus. They may be there because there is viral nucleic acid there, because there is viral protein or they may be there just because the whole nuclear structure is disturbed and in the course of fixation a space appears with normal chromatin. This is probably the basic reason for instance for inclusions following herpes virus infection, it's a fixation artefact really. When you come to the cytoplasm, here again there may be an area in which there is a sort of viral factory set up and this may show differences on staining, or a mass of internal component or something like that which is just accumulated in the cytoplasm in excess, only a small amount of it being incorporated into virus particles. Or again a general degenerative process may be taking place in the cytoplasm because of the way in which its meta-bolism has been disturbed by the virus and this may show up as a definite patch of something in the cell and you say 'ah, there's an inclusion'. So, I think, that in each instance you have got to use the appropriate tests, look for viral protein, look for viral nucleic acid, do electron microscopy if you can and find out what is going on inside the cells. It is a very useful clue to see an inclusion but you cannot say that it is any more than an inclusion until you have investigated it.

Almeida: In answer to Dr Harriman. I think this business of identi-fication of inclusions is terribly important, particularly in SSPE. We have debated the idea that there may be an incomplete virus and it would be very nice to get specific antigen and specific antiserum for the whole virus, for the internal component, perhaps for the haemagglutinin, so that we really could look and see if the trouble in transmissibility or isolation of the virus is because the vast majority of the virus in these specimens is incomplete.

MacCallum: I think Dr Udall has the floor for the next question.

Udall: Just a comment really. I have discussed the subject already with Dr Dayan but I would like to draw attention to some similarities between subacute sclerosing panencephalitis and dog distemper, in which there are very similar inclusion bodies in oligodendrocytes and also the demyelination is very similar indeed to that which Dayan and others have shown. So I am looking forward to a collaboration in this respect.

PARRY: May I just answer, or attempt to answer the question that Professor Calvin asked. I personally am delighted that he can see no incompatibility between our two hypotheses concerning the aetiology of Scrapie because we have been trying to work to this end for the last 10 years. We are of course immensely interested to know whether the transmissible Scrapie agent would enter the genome of the goat. There is some work by Pattison on the experimental disease in goats and in breeding trials I think that he was unable to show any transfer. We have felt that it would be much better to try and use sheep in which the disease is natural—we should have a better chance. We have been doing this but initially I do not think that the genotypes we were using were good enough and the results were not clear cut. We are, at this moment, repeating it with the known susceptible genotypes that we have to hand.

URICH: Dr Webb is still waiting for an answer regarding relationship of astrocytes and oligodendrocytes and I quite agree with him that we have made far too much of differentiation between them. I do not subscribe to the theory that one is a more mature cell than the other. I think they are both equally mature and I will go as far as to say that they are a neuroglial cell in a different state of functional differentiation. I do not think I will be prepared to go any further in the present state of knowledge.

HUGHES: In answer to Dr Webb, I saw a few weeks ago in New York, an electronmicrograph taken by Hirano of an oligodendrocyte and I think it is the first complete electronmicrograph of this cell in a mammal that has ever been seen. It showed the relationship between the nucleus, the cytoplasm around the nucleus, and the bridge of cytoplasm to the whorl around the axon cylinder. This evidence convinces me that the cell we know as the oligodendrocyte has a supportive role to central myelin analogous to the relationship of the Schwann cell to peripheral myelin. I do not think that the mammalial astrocyte has ever been shown to have a similar ultrastructure to that I have described in the oligodendrocyte. I should be most reluctant to accept this idea that oligodendrocytes and astrocytes are in most respects identical. It does not accord with my own experience. Of course if you believe that an osteoblast and a fibroblast are the same sort of cell because occasionally fibroblasts appear to mutate into osteoblasts, you may be prepared to believe that the same lack of specificity exists between an astrocyte and oligodendrocyte. But this is not the same as the difference between the structure and function of the mature cell.

WEBB: I am no expert on this but I did look up the literature rather carefully before coming here and I think Peters (1964) has shown by electronmicroscopy the relationship between the oligodendrocytes and astrocytes and Wendell-Smith (1966) showed equally clearly the relation of the astrocyte to this development and I suggest that if Dr Hughes has not seen these papers he might like to have a look at them because I think they are fairly convincing.

OFFORD: An answer and a question. First, the attempt at an answer to Dr Hunter. It is not entirely an assumption that DNA alone can cause transformation. If the DNA of polyoma is extracted, as far as one can tell, pure from the virus leaving everything else behind this has some rather unique physical properties, and the ability to cause transformation follows these unique physical properties. Thus either one must explain the radiation destruction results in the way that Professor Waterson did or to say that some very very small quantity of contaminant has been associated.

The question very quickly is; has anybody in fact started to look for virus-like bodies in tissue from pathological conditions after removing the cellular debris or are they always done just from cell emulsion or tissue emulsion?

ALMEIDA: To answer that perhaps Dr Tyrrell would tell the story of how we found corona virus.

TYRRELL: Well I was brainwashed actually into doing this having been brought up in my earlier virological training to say that until one had concentrated and purified one's virus one should not waste the electronmicroscopist's time. On this occasion I was talking to Mrs Almeida and saying that we had got some new viruses growing in organ cultures and I wished I knew what they were and she said well just bring the organ cultures up to me and I'll tell you. I didn't really believe this so I first gave her some tests consisting of a number of unlabelled specimens in which I had put viruses whose structure I knew perfectly well. I was rather embarrassed to discover that she scored about nine out of ten I think in this test. Having done this we then put into these tests organ cultures of viruses which we knew were there but could not detect directly by any means and we found this interesting structure, the corona virus.

MacCallum: I think that with those comments we will bring the discussion to a close. Dr Tyrrell commenced in what I believe you will all agree was a very lucid fashion yesterday morning and it is appropriate that he should have the last word today. It only remains for me to thank all the participants and say that I hope that all of you have got something out of this meeting. I think the discussion and the questions, both peaceful and belligerent have demonstrated that this has been so, even though originally I had my doubts as to whether there was enough new material to stimulate people to discussion.

Index

RC
327
.V57